SATAN, I'M TAKING BACK MY HEALTH!

by Dr. Jawanza Kunjufu

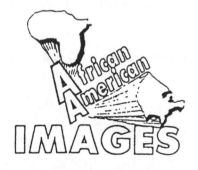

Chicago, Illinois

DEDICATION

This book is dedicated to my late grandmother, Cecil Presentine, my late aunt, Lucille Johnston, both of whom died of cancer in the colon and my mother, Mary Brown, who died October 24, 1998. My mother had the typical American diet and was totally dependent upon the American medical profession for her health. They both failed her. In February of 1998, she experienced discomfort, and after a battery of tests, the conclusion was there was a problem in her gall bladder. Further tests indicated there were numerous gallstones.

The medical profession, rather than asking themselves what caused the development of these gallstones and what naturally can be done to remove them, chose to remove the gallbladder. While removing the gall bladder they also identified malignant tumors and recommended chemotherapy and radiation. For a myriad of reasons I was not in favor of this approach, but because I was not in complete control over the next medical course of action, chemotherapy and radiation were given.

After several months of chemotherapy and radiation which were also destroying her good cells, the medical profession gave up on my mother and told the family it was just a matter of time before she would die. She did six months later. I am thankful my mother was able to achieve God's promise for 70 years, but I know God is not pleased with so many of His children who are dying so early and unnecessarily and not experiencing the quality of life that God wants for them.

The following pages are dedicated to all those who have, as Baby Face Edmonds and Michael Jackson have

iii

coined the song, "Gone Too Soon." The following pages are written to illuminate the kind of life that God wants all of His children to possess. I have high expectations. I no longer use the phrase, if I can just save one person. My desire is to save millions, and I pray this book will achieve all that it was set out to do. May God bless you and keep you all the days of your life.

CONTENTS

INTRODUCTION

I am very excited about this book and I thank you for choosing to read it. I pray that you not only will enjoy this book, but that you will recommend it to others and receive all that God has for your life.

I have been a vegetarian since 1973. The combination of God's grace, a good diet, and regular exercise, has allowed me to never miss a day of work due to illness. I am a Ph.D. not a M.D., nor am I a Naturopath, Chiropractor, or Herbalist. I include these three because unfortunately many Americans are not aware that there are other professions who also can make a major contribution to their health. In a subsequent chapter, you will learn how little medical doctors are trained in the area of nutrition, which I think is paramount to your health.

What I do believe with a Ph.D. is that I have a degree in critical thinking skills. If you've read my other 18 books, you will notice there is a tremendous range in the subjects that I tackle. I am not afraid to write a book on education, values, peer pressure economics, history, fiction, male/female relationships, or religion. I believe Philippians 4:13 "I can do all things through Christ who strengthens me." Over the past year, I have literally read every health book and medical journal to understand the wide range of thought in this massive field of health care.

My desire is not to convert anyone to become a vegetarian. My concern is that I would like for you to live longer. I would like for you to enjoy life to the fullest. I've noticed in our building (the bookstore is on the second floor and our publishing company has its offices on the first floor) that for many of our customers it is a tremendous challenge walking up several stairs to the bookstore. Many of these people are under 40 years of age. People not only are dying earlier than ever before, but they are not living life to the fullest. I want you to be full of energy and vitality.

What makes this book *Satan, I'm Taking Back My Health* so unique in my opinion is that I have attempted to combine a Christian perspective with health care. As you review the Contents page, there is a wide array of chapters, but first meditate on the following anecdotes. They mirror the chapters.

ANECDOTES

1. You are what you eat.

2. You are what you don't eliminate.

3. You are what you drink.

4. Man does not die from guns, he kills himself at the kitchen table with his knife.

5. You are as young as your arteries.

6. Health equals wealth.

7. It is not how long you live, but how you feel while you're living.

8. Do you live to eat or do you eat to live?

9. A civilization is only as strong as its soil.

10. Refined sugar is killing the human race.

11. Pigs eat their own mess so what does that say about you?

12. The greatest gifts a parent could give their children are to introduce them to Jesus Christ and teach them to care for their bodies, which house the Holy Spirit.

13. Who is in charge? Your flesh or your spirit?

14. Does your health belong to doctors or God?

15. The larger the waistline, the shorter the lifeline.

16. How many cigarettes can I smoke and avoid lung cancer?

17. Diet or drugs?

18. Women get sicker, men die quicker.

19. Most Americans like their food fast, fried, fat, or frozen.

WHAT DOES GOD SAY?

Deuteronomy 30:19. "I call heaven and earth as witnesses today against you that I have set before you life and death, blessing and cursing, therefore choose life that both you and your descendants may live."

God has given us free will. Satan is real. A subsequent chapter will talk about the role of Satan and the impact that he has had on our health. God has given us an option. We live in a world of blessings and curses. We live in a world where there is good and evil. We live in a world where there is healthy and harmful food. God wants us to choose life.

John 10:10. "The thief does not come except to steal, kill, and to destroy. I have come that they may have life and that they may have life more abundantly."

God wants us to live. God wants us to have life and to have life more abundantly. God does not want us to be sick. God wants our best. He gave us His only son to teach us how to live. God gave us his only begotten Son that we may have life and have life more abundantly. God is not pleased with his children dying of cancer, heart disease, strokes, and diabetes, nor suffering from obesity, arthritis, and rheumatism.

III John 2. "Beloved, I pray that you may prosper in all things and be in health just as your soul prospers."

The Lord wants us to prosper in all areas, but notice he emphasizes health. This should be done to the same level that our soul prospers. The Bible asks us what good is it for man to gain the whole world and to lose his soul? The Word

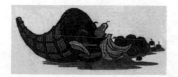
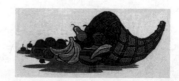

1

teaches, "Seek ye first the Kingdom of God and his righ-
teousness and all these other things shall be added unto it."
The Lord wants first for us to have a relationship with Him.
If you love me you will be my sheep and I will be your shep-
herd and you will hear my voice. Enoch walked with God.
We need to walk with God by obeying His Word.

What has God promised us? Do we have an inheritance? Did our Father leave us a will?

Genesis 12:1–3. "Now the Lord said to Abraham,
get out of your country from your family and from
your father's house to a land that I will show you. I
will make you a great nation. I will bless you and
make your name great, and you shall be a blessing. I
will bless those who bless you and I will curse him
who curses you and in you all the families of the earth
shall be blessed. "

Romans 8:16–17. "The Spirit himself bears witness
with our spirit that we are children of God and if children then heirs, heirs of God and joint heirs with
Christ. If indeed we suffer with him that we may also
be glorified together."

We have a covenant. The same covenant that God
gave to Abraham is the same covenant that God gave to
Abraham's descendants. We are Abraham's descendants.
Many of us were unaware of that covenant. Many of us have
not taken ownership of our inheritance. We are heirs to the
throne. We are joint heirs with Jesus Christ to all that our
Father has for us. The earth is the Lord's and the fullness
thereof. All that God has belongs to us. Every good and
perfect gift belongs to us. Many of us are walking around as
ill paupers, rather than healthy kings and queens. God wants
the best for us, or He would not have appointed us heirs.

Can you imagine a wealthy parent developing a will and including people they don't know, don't like, and don't have a relationship with? Parents who are millionaires are very deliberate about their wills. How unfortunate that many of us do not realize our inheritance. The government reports there are numerous inheritances where heirs have not made claims. They didn't know the inheritance existed. The government has been unable to locate them and after a period of time, the inheritance belongs to the government. This is happening to many Christians.

Psalm 91:16. "With long life I will satisfy him."

God wants us to have long life. God is not pleased when His babies die at birth nor is He pleased when His youth are victims of homicide. God is not pleased when His children die of diseases before they become parents or grandparents. The scripture reminds us, God wants us to have a long life. The following scriptures define how long that life could be.

Genesis 5:27. "So all the days of Methuselah were 969 years and he died."

Genesis 6:3. "And the Lord said my spirit shall not strive with man forever for he is indeed flesh yet his days shall be 120 years."

Psalm 90:10. "The days of our lives are 70 years and if by reason of strength they are 80 years."

God reminds us that with long life I will satisfy him. Our purpose in life is to glorify Him, to bring glory to Him. He wants to give us long life. Methuselah was able to benefit from that promise and live 969 years. With Satan and sin rampant, our life was scaled down to 120 years and further reduced to 70 and 80 with strength. At the very least it should be 70 years, but it should be 70 good years. It should not be in the latter years that you can barely walk, and your body is filled with pain and drugs. God wants us to die of old age and disease free.

I Corinthians, 3:16–17 and 6:19–20. "Or do you not know that your body is the temple of the Holy Spirit who is in you whom you have from God and you are not your own. For you were bought at a price therefore glorify God in your body and in your spirit which are God's." Our body is His temple. We have been bought with a price. Jesus paid the ultimate sacrifice for us. The least we could do is when people see us they see God. Look at yourself for a moment. When people look at your body, do they see God? When people look at you, do they see life, vitality, vigor, and energy? Or do they see someone tired, run down, overweight, sluggish, and out of shape? Our body is His temple. We are not our own. Can you imagine that, we are not our own? Our health and body do not belong to doctors. We belong to Him. He is the potter and we are the clay. The Holy Spirit needs a better place to reside. The Holy Spirit does not need to live in a shell filled with arthritis, rheumatism, diabetes, high blood pressure, heart disease, and cancer. The Holy Spirit deserves better.

Proverbs 23:2-3. "Put a knife to your throat if you are a man given to appetite. Do not desire his delicacies for they are deceptive food." In the anecdotes, I mentioned that man does not die, he kills himself. We kill ourselves at the dinner table. We have a much greater chance of dying at the dinner table than from a gun, an automobile, or a nuclear weapon. Man kills himself with his knife and fork. Man kills himself with delicacies and deceptive foods that we will talk about in the chapter on Satan. You are what you eat. We have a responsibility to God because our body is His temple, to push away from the table.

I know it is hard. I love to eat and some of the delicacies and deceptive foods that I have fallen guilty to are french fries and potato chips. I could avoid making that statement and make it appear that I never eat anything wrong. I could deceive you, and tell you all I do is eat fruits and vegetables, drink eight glasses of water, breathe good air, exercise daily, and will live as long as Methuselah. Many people will hope, because of ego and sin, that I will experience an illness. This will allow them to rationalize that if I could not practice what I preach, how could they.

Our eyes should not be on the preacher, our eyes should be on Christ. If we are honest with each other, what we really are trying to do when we point a finger at someone, is make an opportunity to avoid doing what we know is correct. We all have weaknesses, but it does not make the weakness acceptable. My weaknesses should not be your opportunity and rationale to continue to do what you want. God does not want us to be gluttons. God does not want us to be overweight. Please don't misquote me; that does not mean that God does not love us. God's love for us is unconditional, but it does not negate what He says in His word. We are to avoid deceptive food and delicacies and we are to monitor our appetite and put the knife and fork down. Not only does God want us to put the knife and fork down, but the Bible is filled with scriptures that talk about the value of fasting. Our Lord and Savior Jesus fasted on numerous occasions and often for forty days. David fasted, Daniel fasted, Samuel and Ezra fasted. Numerous people in the Bible fasted. It is not only good for the body, but allows us to become closer to God.

Food becomes a major part of the day. It often takes us away from God. Many of us eat so much that we are not convinced that we can skip one meal and not be completely overwhelmed by hunger pains. Fasting allows the body to rest and heal. Digestion is very demanding on the body. The following chapter on the body will illuminate the demands of digestion. That can explain why many of us after we eat fall asleep. The body is overwhelmed by the work involved. Ironically, for those people who have not fasted, they don't realize that fasting will actually give them energy. The energy that was being used to digest food is now being used to achieve other objectives. The term breakfast—break the fast—should be considered. You don't break a fast with bacon, sausage, eggs, potatoes, and biscuits.

> Proverbs 20:1. "Wine is a mocker, strong drink is a brawler and whoever is led astray by it is not wise."

> Proverbs 21:17. "He who loves wine and oil will not be rich."

> Proverbs 23:31–32. "Do not look on the wine when it is red when it sparkles in the cup when it swirls around smoothly, at the last it bites like a serpent and stings like a vapor. Your eyes will see strange things and your heart will utter perverse things."

> First Corinthians, 6:9–10. "Do you not know that the unrighteous will not inherit the Kingdom of God. Do not be deceived, not the fornicators, nor idolaters, not adulterers, nor homosexuals, nor sodomites, nor thieves, nor covetous, nor drunkards, nor revelers, nor extortioners will inherit the Kingdom of God."

God is very clear about alcohol and wine. Many people make a mockery and simply have communion every day of the week during the entire day. Satan will use research from France that a glass of wine is good for cholesterol. God is clear about drunkards, wine, and strong spirits. We are to abstain. Not only is it not good for you and your holy temple, but if you become a drunkard, you will be denied entrance into the Kingdom of God. Now let's be honest, can wine do you like Jesus? Liquor like the Lord? How unfortunate that Satan has so many people making the wrong choice.

Remember God wants you to choose life. He has placed before you blessings and curses, but he wants you to choose life. He wants you to have life and have life more abundantly. If you love me keep my commandments says the Lord. God is not the author of confusion. Satan is the author of confusion. God gave you the spirit of discernment.

Many people take scriptures out of context. People who believe in white supremacy refer to Ephesians 6:5 where slaves should obey their masters, but if you read further, God also reminds masters how they are to treat the slaves. There are men who have never been to church, but through osmosis learned Ephesians 5:22 where it says women should submit and obey their husbands. If you read further, it also reminds men that they are to submit to one another, and the man is to love his wife as much as God loved the church and as much as he loves his own body.

There are many male pastors who take scriptures out of context and say that women should be silent in the church. Women cannot be deacons, officials, or pastors. If you read Romans 16, Priscilla was an officer in the Church. If you read Galatians 3:28, God is not a respecter of male or female, Jews or Gentile; we are all one in Christ Jesus. We are not to take scriptures out of context. God is not the author of confusion. It would be very easy for me to push my vegetarian diet and support it biblically.

Genesis:1:29 "I have given you every green herb that yields seed which is on the face of all the earth and every tree whose fruit yields seeds; to you it shall be for food."

Daniel 1:12–15. "Please test your servants for ten days, and let them give us vegetables to eat and water to drink. Then let our appearance be examined before you, and the appearance of the young men who eat the portion of the king's delicacies; and as you see fit, so deal with your servants. So he consented with them in this matter, and tested them ten days. And at the end of ten days their features appeared better and fatter in flesh than all the young men who ate the portion of the king's delicacies." This is called the "Daniel Fast" which I recommend and live by.

Throughout the Bible, God talks about the importance of fruits and vegetables, the significance of herbs and yet if you read:

I Timothy, 4:4–5. "For every creature of God is good and nothing is to be refused if it is received with thanksgiving, for it is sanctified by the word of God and prayer." Romans, 14:2, "For one believes he may eat all things, but he who is weak eats only vegetables."

God is not the author of confusion and yet it appears that as a vegetarian I am weak in the faith. It appears that all food is edible based on your level of faith and if it is received with thanksgiving and prayer.

Leviticus 11:2–7. "Speak to the children of Israel saying these the animals which you may eat among all the animals that are on the earth. Among the animals whatever divides the hoof having cloven hoofs and chewing the cud, that you may eat. Nevertheless, these you should not eat. Among those that chew the cud or those that have cloven hoofs. The camel because he chews the cud but does not have cloven hoofs is unclean to you. The rock hyrax because it chews the cud but does not have cloven hoofs is unclean to you, the hare because it chews the cud but does not have cloven hoofs is unclean to you, and the swan though it divides the hoof having cloven hoofs it does not chew the cud is unclean to you. Their flesh you shall not eat and their carcasses you shall not touch. They are not clean to you."

Deuteronomy, 14:3–21 reinforces the 11th Chapter of Leviticus. It seems that you can use the Bible to support whatever diet you want. God has rules in Deuteronomy and Leviticus about some foods that we should not eat, but a person could use the scripture in I Timothy and Romans to override those scriptures because all food is blessed if it is received with thanksgiving and prayer.

A vegetarian could rationalize their position with Genesis 1:29 and the Daniel diet and yet be told he has weak faith in Romans 14. Meat eaters can rationalize that their diet is supported not only by I Timothy and Romans, but all the other animals that God said were okay to eat. So how do we reconcile all these scriptures and believe that God is not the author of confusion? I'm glad you asked.

Isaiah 55:2. "Eat that which is good."

Hosea 4:8. "My people suffer from lack of knowledge." II Timothy, 2:15 reminds us, "To study to show thyself approved, rightly dividing the word of God." God gives us a discerning spirit. Eat that which is good, not tastes good, but is good for His temple. All of us have to ask ourselves before we eat, is this what God wants us to have? For meat eaters, take a trip to a meat factory and then ask yourself is that what God wants me to consume?

Clean chitterlings and then ask yourself is this good? Cook chitterlings and smell the stench, and ask yourself is this good? Read the labels on the food that you eat, and ask yourself is this something I want to put into my body which houses the Holy Spirit?

The next chapter is on your beautiful body, that it is fearfully and wonderfully made. Let's look at how God made you, made you so wonderfully and the plans God has for your life.

YOUR WONDERFUL BODY

Psalm 139:13–14. "For you formed my inward parts. You covered me in my mother's womb. I will praise you for I am fearfully and wonderfully made."

Matthew 10:30. "But the very hairs of your head are all numbered."

When I talk to people, many of whom possess bachelors, masters, and doctorate degrees yet, many have little understanding and knowledge about their body. It was as if attending elementary and high school science classes only taught about the moon, stars and plants, but did not give them a firm understanding of their bodies. What is the purpose of your liver? What is the purpose of your kidneys? What percentage of your body is made of water? What do you know about your cells? What is the purpose of the gallbladder and pancreas? What is the difference between the small intestine, large intestine, and colon? Where is the thyroid and what is its purpose?

For most of us we are unable to successfully answer those questions and it's not our fault. We have been trained, but not educated. A person truly educated knows *whose* he is, *who* he is, his purpose in life, and lastly understands his body and how to keep it at maximum proficiency.

In a subsequent chapter, *The Doctor Said!,* many of us not only do not possess a good understanding of the body, but have no desire, and have relinquished our health to the medical profession and the pharmaceutical industry. This is one of the major reasons for this book. God gave our bodies to us and it is our responsibility to maintain them.

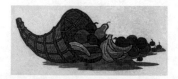
11
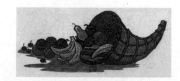

The objective of this chapter is to give you a better understanding of how fearfully and wonderfully you are made. Many people refer to God as the creator, the higher force, the man upstairs, but His name is Jesus and after reading this chapter, I can't fathom that an atheist would surmise that their body was constructed accidentally. Our bodies truly are a gift from God and when you understand and believe the Giver you can't help but become more grateful and appreciative. I don't believe it's an accident that the same 103 minerals that are found in the earth are also found in your body. Isn't that amazing that our bodies parallel the earth?

In the following chapter on *Satan,* we will talk about soil erosion and how many of the minerals and vitamins that were in the earth are absent. God intended for our bodies to parallel the earth. Our bodies come from the earth and they will return to the earth. Note I said our bodies, not our spirits. For those who are saved, our spirits will have everlasting life in heaven. Because our bodies parallel the earth, it is our responsibility to make sure that we consume the 103 minerals and vitamins we so desperately need in order to have vitality. Most of us are not aware of those 103 minerals and vitamins.

In a subsequent chapter, *You Are What You Eat,* we will mention many of those minerals and vitamins in more detail. Suffice to say in this chapter that it is our responsibility each day to make sure that we consume enough vitamin A, B, C, D, E, calcium, potassium, iron, magnesium, zinc and so many more in order to enjoy life to the fullest. Nor do I believe that it is an accident that 80 percent of the earth and our bodies consist of water. Therefore, since a large part of our body consists of water, we should try to consume a minimum of eight glasses daily.

In a subsequent chapter on *Lifestyle and Habits* one obvious reason why we don't consume water is because water is not advertised, while Pepsi, Coca Cola, alcohol, coffee, and numerous other drinks have billion dollar advertising budgets. Many people have been conditioned not to like water. Our bodies have 43 hundred gallons of water. Eighty-three percent of our blood consists of water, 82 percent of our kidneys consist of water, 75 percent of our muscles consist of water, 74 percent of the brain, and 22 percent of our bones are made of water.

It should be obvious that if we do not consume an adequate amount of water, it not only affects the quality and circulation of our blood, but it affects the functioning of our kidneys, muscles, bones, and our brain. How unfortunate that many Americans are dependent on a dialysis machine for their kidneys. All that could have been circumvented had they given their kidneys an adequate amount of water.

Our bodies have five major systems: skeletal, respiratory, circulatory, nervous, and excretory. Our bodies have 630 muscles and 206 bones, and 60 trillion cells. Our 206 bones are connected to each other by joints. At the end of each bone is cartilage. The bones are held together by strong stretching bands called ligaments. One of our 630 muscles is the brain. The brain weighs approximately three pounds. The brain via nerve cells can transmit over 1,000 nerve impulses every second. For those who marvel at computers, specifically the hardware and their ability to store data, there is no comparison between man-made hardware and the awesomeness of God and what He did with three pounds. He gave you the best hardware, unlimited memory.

God continues to show His brilliance in the circulatory system. Our heart pumps 30 million times per year. Our heart pumps 250,000 gallons of blood over a lifetime.

Our bodies consist of six quarts of blood. The arteries carry blood away from the heart, and the veins take blood to the heart. Blood flows through our entire bodies in less than two minutes. Our arteries break down into small blood vessels called capillaries. The red blood cells carry oxygen from the lungs to all cells. Our white blood cells protect the body from disease. In the anecdotes, I mentioned you are as healthy as your arteries. If they are clogged with toxins and cholesterol you are at risk. One of every two Americans will suffer from a heart attack. There is a relationship between blood pressure, strokes, and heart attacks. You are as healthy as your blood. You are as healthy as the flow of the blood through your veins and arteries. Clogged arteries and veins will put an unnecessary burden on your heart.

Just as God gave the children of Israel new manna each day, He gives us new mercies each day; He does the same with our bodies. We have 60 trillion cells and 80 million blood cells die every second, and amazingly the same number are born. We receive new blood every 90 days. We receive new cells for our organs every 12 months and no cell is older than seven years. Cell regeneration is another gift from God. It is never too late to change our diet and experience the God of a "second chance."

The liver is the largest organ in our body after the skin. It weighs between 42 and 53 ounces and has over 500 functions. It metabolizes all foods. Oftentimes, when you finish eating you feel warm. Digesting food takes a great degree of work and creates heat. Three pints of blood flow through the liver per minute. It stores vitamins and minerals. The liver filters harmful chemicals and creates bile which breaks down fat and removes cholesterol. It stores blood for emergencies. It maintains the water balance in the body. The liver eliminates unnecessary hormones. Why would anyone intentionally harm their liver? Why would anyone drink liquor and consume food that will harm if not destroy the liver knowing the liver has over 500 functions?

The bile that the liver produces is stored in the gallbladder, which sends bile to the intestines for digestion and removes cholesterol from the body. My mother died of gallbladder cancer. Her gallbladder was filled with numerous stones which were the result of an excessive amount of cholesterol. A greater understanding of the function of the liver and gallbladder could have saved her. In a subsequent chapter on *Healing* we will look at different strategies to remove gallstones and malignant tumors. There are other strategies beside surgery, radiation, and chemotherapy.

When you hear the word cholesterol, what comes to your mind? Would you be surprised if I told you that you produce 80 percent of the cholesterol in your body? Not all cholesterol is bad. The body needs cholesterol in order to function. Cholesterol is divided into two categories: HDL and LDL. HDL takes cholesterol out of the arteries and distributes it to other organs in the body for its own function. HDL is good cholesterol. LDL deposits cholesterol in arteries creating plaque. LDL cholesterol is detrimental to our bodies.

Another major organ is the kidney. Kidneys filter waste products from the blood at 1200 milliliters per minute. If the kidneys are not working properly, then we become a walking cesspool with contaminated toxic blood. Your health and vitality can be measured by the quality of your blood.

The function of the pancreas is to produce insulin to balance the sugar in our bodies. It also provides digestive juices for proper elimination. In a subsequent chapter on *The Big Debate*, we will look at diabetes, diet, specifically sugar, carbohydrates, insulin, and the excess work on the pancreas. There has been much concern about the pancreas, diabetes, sugar consumption, obesity, the protein diet, and carbohydrates. I wanted to reserve an entire chapter to look at these issues.

Many Americans are living longer, but the quality of their life is lacking. Many Americans are tired and fatigued. One major reason is their thyroid gland. The thyroid affects metabolism, energy level, and weight. All of us need to learn more about the thyroid and the food it needs to operate at maximum efficiency.

The last three organs that we want to review are the small intestine, large intestine, and colon. The small intestine is 25 feet long, but its width is the size of a dime. Nutrients are absorbed in the small intestine. Substances it cannot use are passed to the large intestine, which is only five feet long, but three inches wide. One of the major functions of the large intestine is to remove water from the food creating solid waste matter which will be distributed to the colon for elimination.

There is a major relationship between the quality of the food we eat and the efficiency and productivity of the small intestine, large intestine, and colon. Many natural healers, i.e. chiropractors, naturopaths, herbalists, and colon therapists feel the state of our health can be determined by the quality of the colon. One of the anecdotes was you are what you do not eliminate. I reserved an entire chapter so that we can further understand the importance of the small intestine, large intestine, and colon and the significance of the food we consume.

I hope this chapter on your body has given you a better understanding on how wonderfully you are made. God has every hair numbered. You are not an accident. Your body is amazing and we suffer from a lack of knowledge. We need to study to show thyself approved. Unfortunately, Satan also knows how wonderfully you are made and in the following chapter we will understand that Satan comes to kill, steal, and to destroy our bodies.

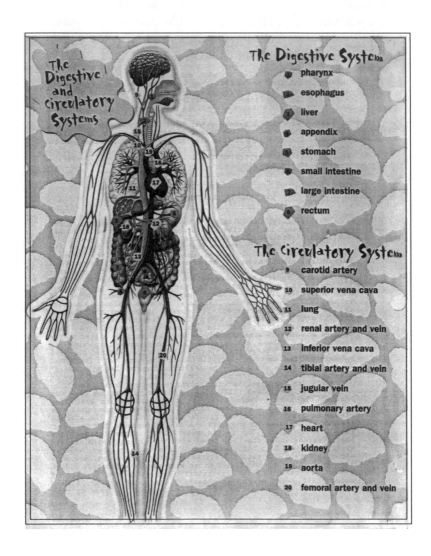

THE ROLE OF SATAN

Thirty-five million Americans suffer from depression. Heart disease is the number one killer in America. Two million Americans die annually. It was unheard of in the early 1900s. One million people are diagnosed with cancer annually; 500,000 die. Two hundred and fifty thousand American males are diagnosed with prostate cancer; 40,000 die annually. Fifty seven thousand Americans die of colon cancer. Six hundred and fifty thousand Americans annually are diagnosed with a disease in their gallbladder.

One of every three Americans will die of cancer. Fifty million Americans smoke, thirty-three percent of all men smoke and twenty-eight percent of all women and the latter are rising. The popular commercial stated, "You've come a long way baby." Women can now kill themselves at the same magnitude as men. Smoking also contributes to heart disease. Seventy percent of all smokers want to quit. One third try annually and only three percent are successful.

Motor accidents are the third leading killer for Americans. Liquor is a major contributor. Diabetes is the third leading killer among African Americans and the sixth leading killer for Americans overall. Fifty percent of Americans have a blood sugar disorder. Thirty million American males are impotent, which translates into one of every six males suffering from this disease. Almost all alcoholics become impotent because alcohol destroys testosterone, the male sex hormone. Forty million Americans suffer from arthritis. Thirty-five percent have arthritis after age thirty-five. Two-hundred and seventeen thousand Americans have kidney failure and are on dialysis. Twenty percent of the elderly suffer from incontinence and fifty percent of elders in nursing homes are suffering from this dreaded illness. One of

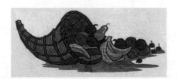 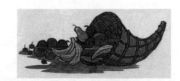

19

every eight women will have breast cancer. Thirty percent of Americans are obese and they spend $32 billion annually trying to lose weight. Eight thousand Americans die of heroin, 12,000 of cocaine, 100,000 of liquor, and 435,000 from cigarettes.[1]

When I give workshops to youth, I ask them which drug do they think kills the most. Invariably, they choose heroin or cocaine. They underestimate Satan, who does not start us on the hard stuff first. He starts with liquor and cigarettes. As you can see from the above figures, it really isn't necessary for Satan to move us to heroin and cocaine when he can kill us with liquor and cigarettes.

Many people think when they hear the word addictions, that only encompasses heroin or cocaine. In actuality, the four drugs that are most addictive to Americans are sugar, caffeine, alcohol, and nicotine. One hundred years ago Americans only consumed four pounds of sugar, today Americans consume 155 pounds![2]

In the previous chapter, we mentioned that our bodies parallel the earth and both consist of 103 minerals and vitamins. One of the major problems in our society is that the soil does not have the same nutrients it had 100 years ago. The American soil had 21 inches of topsoil. Our minerals and vitamins were in the topsoil. Today, it has less than six inches. We are losing seven billion tons of topsoil annually. Eighty-five percent of that loss is due to livestock. Americans' excessive desire to consume meat has become very costly. The amount of acreage allocated for livestock is destroying the top soil needed by humans. We are losing four million acres of land annually due to livestock. The remaining fifteen percent of our topsoil loss is due to industrial waste, fertilizer, and pesticides. One of the anecdotes was that a civilization is only as strong as its soil. America is dying due to topsoil erosion. There has been a 400 percent increase in meat consumption over the past century.[3]

In Genesis 2:16, God lets man know what is available to him, what is good for him and only has one restriction. "The Lord commanded the man saying of every tree of the garden, you may freely eat but of the tree of knowledge of good and evil, you shall not eat for in the day that you eat of it, you shall surely die." Unfortunately, man has not kept God's desire for his diet. We read in Genesis 1:29, God has given man every herb for food.

Satan is real and many of us underestimate him. In Genesis 3:1–7. "The woman said to the serpent, we may eat the fruit of the trees of the garden, but of the fruit of the tree which is in the midst of the garden God had said, you shall not eat it nor shall you touch it lest you die. Then the serpent said to the woman, you will not surely die for God knows that in the day you eat of it, your eyes will be open and you will be like God knowing good and evil. So when the woman saw that the tree was good for food and it was pleasant to the eyes and the tree desirable to make one wise, she took of its fruit and ate. She also gave to her husband and he ate." It has been downhill ever since for the human population. Satan continues to kill, steal, and destroy. He only has power that we give him. He is the originator of lies, a deceiver, and author of confusion. Esau lost his birthright because he was controlled by food.

Have you ever had a desire to do the right thing and ended up doing the wrong thing? Have you ever promised yourself that you were not going to not eat as much during the holidays and yet you consumed more than you could ever imagine? Have you ever been in a situation where you told yourself you were not going to succumb to peer pressure and drink and smoke and yet in the heat of the moment, you did it anyway?

In Romans, 7:15–25. "For what I am doing I do not understand. For what I will do, that I do not practice for what I hate that I do. If then I do what I will not to do, I agree with the law that is good but now it is no longer I who do it but sin that dwells in me. For I know that in me, that is in my flesh, nothing good dwells but for to will is present with me but how to perform what is good, I do not find. For the good that I will to do, I do not do but the evil, I will not to do that I practice. Now if I do what I will not to do, it is no longer I who do it but sin that dwells in me. I find then a law that evil is present with me, the one who wills to do good for I delight in the law of God according to the inward man but I see another law in my members warring against the law of the mind and bringing me into captivity to the law of sin which is in my members old wretched man that I am, who will deliver me from this body of death? I thank God through Jesus Christ our Lord so then with the mind, I might self serve the law of God but with the flesh, the law of sin."

We must die to the flesh. We must discipline our flesh. We must not allow our flesh to kill us at the kitchen table. One of Satan's most effective tricks is "delayed consequences." I sincerely believe that if people became immediately addicted to liquor, cigarettes, and cocaine, then people would be more careful about using those drugs. If there was an immediate reaction to the consumption of pork, ice cream, sugar, donuts, and other popular American foods then people would curtail if not eliminate them from their diet. Unfortunately, the body's reaction to these items is not immediate. It is over a period of time. Consequently, people assume they can violate God's law without consequences. In this era of sexual promiscuity, if every time you had sex out of marriage, you encountered a sexually transmitted disease, or became a victim of HIV, or conceived I think people would be less promiscuous. Satan leads us to believe we can sin without consequences.

I had the opportunity to sit next to a very sick woman on an airplane. She was unable to lock her seatbelt or let down her tray for her meal, and had a difficult time feeding herself. I tried to assist her in every way possible. She reminded me of my mother, and the scripture says, "what you do unto the least of these, you also do unto me." She broke my heart later when she said, "I want a cigarette." I asked her, "But what about your health?" She said, "Cigarettes don't hurt me."

The first thing that came to my mind is that we struggle not against flesh and blood, but principalities and rulers in high places. That was a demon speaking to me, an evil spirit inside of her body that had led her to believe in spite of all of her ailments that cigarettes would not hurt her. She had probably smoked before she boarded the plane and was looking forward to landing to smoke again. At this late hour, Satan still controlled her.

Another one of Satan's tricks is "moderation." He convinces most of us that even if the research says that this particular food or drug has harmful effects, if you only consume a little, it will not hurt you. A little adultery, a little fornication, a little reefer, a little cocaine, just a couple drinks, just a couple cigarettes, pork only for breakfast, and fried foods once a day will not hurt you.

Another one of Satan's tricks is "exceptions to the rules." The research shows one of every three American smokers will suffer from lung cancer. Satan responds, and tells you two of every three will not. People love to tell me about their relative who lived to be 100 while smoking, drinking, and eating fried pork. How naive to compare someone who lived in the early 1900s who consumed less sugar and meat, consumed a greater number of vitamins and minerals due to greater topsoil, ate less food that was processed and packaged in boxes and cans, who walked three miles to school and work. We have the nerve to compare ourselves to that person! Another trick of the devil.

Another popular strategy of Satan is using "conflicting research" to confuse the public. Almost daily Americans are told about another food that is harmful. One day you hear that red meat is detrimental; several days later you hear that chicken and turkey are harmful. Several days later you hear the mercury level for fish is toxic. You then decide maybe I should become a vegetarian until a study shows that pesticides on fruits and vegetables have increased. You had just given up on alcohol and then a study from France reports that a glass of wine after dinner is actually good for the blood and you'll have less chance of a heart attack. Alcohol increases breast cancer by 50 percent. Foods advertised as "no cholesterol" are actually high in fat. Foods advertised "low fat" are actually high in sugar and calories. The American public then becomes so confused and frustrated that many people say, well you have to die of something and so I choose to die of this, and Satan again has gotten another one to fall for his tricks.

I remember my late uncle who died of lung cancer was told by his doctor that if he did not give up cigarettes he would be dead in less than three months. My uncle looked the doctor dead in the eye and said, "I would feel dead if I did not have a cigarette." That was a demon coming out of my uncle. Satan had convinced him that cigarettes were synonymous with life. Had my uncle known 30 years prior that his nicotine addiction would make him say a statement like that he never would have smoked.

The Bible reminds us, "Thou shall have no other God before Him." Unfortunately, many of us have made food our God. For many of us there are certain types of food that have become so addictive that we cannot live without them. There are some Americans that cannot have a meal without meat or cannot go to bed without ice cream. Let me ask you an honest question. Do you live to eat or do you eat to live? Is there a food that controls you? Is there a food that you cannot do without? I would like for you to fast on that food. I would like for you to take control of your life. I would like for you to control Satan. Just as Jesus fasted for 40 days, I would like for you for the next 40 days not to consume that food that has you addicted. Words of confession lead to possession. Tell yourself that the food that had you in bondage is disgusting. If you give that food a negative connotation you can break the yoke. After 40 days, you will no longer be addicted.

The last trick that I want to share in this chapter is that many Americans believe they are living longer. Throughout this book, I am going to point out that beyond the issue of longevity, God reminds us that He came to give us life and to give us life more abundantly. Satan has so impressed us with longevity that we are not looking at the quality of life. My mother told my sister and me that she did not want to live on a respirator. She was very much aware that the medical profession had the ability to keep her alive on respirators, fed intravenously, and addicted to medicine.

This book is about the *quality* of life. Satan has not only lied to us about the quality of life, but its longevity. Many Americans believe they are living longer than ever before. Figures don't lie, but liars figure. Now it is true, life expectancy over this past century has grown from a mere 47 years of age to 73 years of age, but that is not due to better diet and exercise. The most important factor that has contributed to almost a 30 year increase in life expectancy is our almost elimination of infant mortality, tuberculosis, and pneumonia.[4]

Let me illustrate this in a simple mathematical example. You have two people, they were both born in 1930. One lived to the year 2000 and the other died at birth. If the world's population only consisted of those two people then the life expectancy would be 35 years of age. If the second person did not die at birth and had lived even to 60 years of age, then the life expectancy would dramatically increase from 35 years to now 65 years. It does not mean the first person is living longer. We are living longer, but that is primarily due to the reduction of those three illnesses and specifically infant mortality rate. Americans are only living 18 months longer than they did at the turn of the century, if you exclude people who died of infant mortality, tuberculosis, and pneumonia.

We have new illnesses that Americans are dying of that did not exist to this magnitude at the turn of the 20th century. In the early 1900s one of 33 Americans died of cancer, but today it is one of three. One of every two will die of heart disease, which was unheard of in the early 1900s. God does not want you to die of cancer and heart disease. God wants you to die of old age. God does not want you to die before his promise of 70 years, 80 with strength, and possibly 120 years. God not only wants you to live a long life so that you can satisfy Him, He wants to improve the quality of your life. He does not want you to suffer with arthritis, rheumatism, diabetes, impotence, and high blood pressure.

Satan has made us ignorant of our bodies. It is one thing not to know, but it is worse when you don't care to know. We not only lack the knowledge about our bodies and the foods that we need to consume, but many of us do not care.

How much do you love God? Do you trust him? Do you believe in His word? Do you believe that He came to give you life and to give you life more abundantly? Do you believe that He wants you to prosper in all things including your health just as your soul prospers? Do you believe that He has a covenant with you and that you are a joint heir with Jesus and an heir to the throne? Do you believe that Jesus rose with all power in His hands? If you believe that then you also know Satan only has the power we give him. Satan's power is in rumors, deceptions, and lies. The Bible reminds us that God wants us to choose life. He wants us to choose life over sugar. God wants us to chose life over caffeine. God wants us to choose life over alcohol, nicotine, cocaine, heroin, and pork. Is there anything that controls you? Do you have an addiction?

You have been purchased with a price. You do not belong to an addiction. We struggle not against flesh and blood, but principalities and rulers in high places. We struggle against those addictions. Use the Holy Spirit, scriptures, and prayer. These are the weapons of our warfare for pulling down strongholds. Use these gifts from God to remove burdens and destroy yokes.

In a powerful book by George Malkmus, *Why Christians Get Sick*, the author points out that Christians seem to be no better than any other segment of the population concerning illness and disease. Satan loves this. Many Christians are passive about their health and don't want to take responsibility by exercising and diet. A popular joke is that you can tell if a person is saved—they gain weight and look less attractive. Many Christians give up on their earthly life and concentrate solely on their eternal life. Some rationalize their illness due to their sins and God's will.[5]

In the following chapter, we will look at how our lifestyle has affected our health.

LIFESTYLE AND HABITS

I would like for you to answer the following questions: How much water did you drink today? Earlier we mentioned that your body is 80 percent water and it is imperative that we drink a minimum of eight glasses of water. Unfortunately in the American lifestyle most of us do not drink an adequate amount of water. Many people tell me they do not like water. They do not like the taste. Satan would have us to believe that Pepsi, Coca Cola, and 7-Up are better than water. When was the last time you saw water advertised? What compounds the problem is that many who understand the need for water, live in cities where the water is polluted.

Another trick from Satan is contaminated water. We are responsible to find clean water and drink eight glasses. The solution is not the elimination of water or the replacement of water with pop. The answer is either in buying a filter that will remove lead, fluoride, and other harmful elements, buying distilled, or other forms of bottled water, or boiling water.

The American lifestyle, which consumes very little water, has dire consequences on our overall health. The quality of our blood, kidneys, liver, small intestine, large intestine, and colon are affected. Start the day with a glass of water. On your job, try to consume water. One of the ways to reduce food consumption is to drink a glass of water twenty minutes before eating. If you exercise, that will encourage you to drink water. Before retiring for the evening, consume what is necessary to achieve your eight glasses. I have found the size of my container helps to achieve my goal, and drinking while commuting.

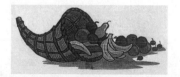
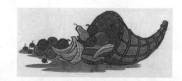

29

This may seem shocking to you, but we are not to eat and drink simultaneously. Our digestive system becomes overwhelmed and confused when we combine liquids with solids. Our pancreas provides different digestive juices for liquids and solids. When the two are combined, the system either shuts off or it chooses to digest the liquids because they are simpler, and solid food is delayed. Depending upon what we have eaten, many times it is not digested at all and petrifies in the system. One of the reasons why so many of us eat and drink simultaneously is because the food that we eat is so dead and dry that we need liquid in order to "wash it down."

I wonder how much liquid it takes to wash down watermelon, cantaloupe, grapefruit, oranges, honeydew melon, lettuce, tomatoes, and cucumbers? I have observed children and adults playing in the summer and becoming thirsty. I know God is sure His children will choose water to quench their thirst. Satan sends the ice cream truck to the park and they buy ice cream and pop, but after consuming it, their body is still craving for the only source that can satisfy their thirst – water!

Hopefully, you will do a better job with the second set of questions. Did you eat anything real today? Did you eat anything that was alive? Did everything you eat come from a box or a can? Did you eat any raw food today? Was everything that you ate today cooked? Can you imagine that many of us have gone the entire day and everything we ate was dead? All the food that we ate was void of minerals and vitamins. Our bodies are alive. Our cells are alive. Cancer is the result of giving dead food to a live body. The consequence is that cells die prematurely. How much live food did your grandparents between the 1900s and the 1940s consume? I wonder between the 1900s and the 1940s, how many

Snickers, bags of potato chips, and bottles of pop did they consume? I wonder how many cans of fruit, and frozen packages of vegetables did they consume?

One major factor driving this change in food consumption is the move from the farm to the city. Over eighty-five percent of the American population now lives in an urban environment and the figure is rising. There are other factors that make this more complex. In an urban environment there is less opportunity to purchase fruits and vegetables. I was sharing with my wife, there is a thirty minute trip between our house and our business. There is not one produce market along the route. We would have to go out of our way in order to buy produce. I remember after a speaking engagement, I asked the driver to stop so I could buy some fruit. We stopped literally at every food mart along the highway and everything in the food mart was dead. If I had asked him to stop to buy candy, potato chips, pop, beer, donuts or cookies that would not have been a problem.

I knew Satan was laughing and God was distraught. I wanted to eat what God made and Satan had made that unavailable. For those who do not value raw food or do not care, they are oblivious to the above. My wife and I were attending a concert one evening and a movie the following day; there is something about a concert, movie, or ballgame that makes you hungry. Try attending one of these events and buying something real. When is the last time you attended a concert, movie, or ball game and had the opportunity to purchase fruit, salad, or vegetable juice? Why is it that at a concert, ball game or the movie theatre, they can provide hot dogs, hamburgers, and nachos but no live food?

Notice I did not say airports, being a frequent flyer, I could write a book on airports and airplanes. They service a slightly higher upscale audience. Most airports are at least willing to provide some fruit and salads. Granted, they are overpriced, but I appreciate their presence. Many vendors tell me the problem is that the fruit spoils due to low demand. I often fly first class and there is a major difference in the quality of meals between first class and coach. In coach, you cannot recognize the food; it has been dead for months. In first class, granted there is steak, but before steak, there is a full salad, with good lettuce.

Notice I did not say a salad with iceberg lettuce, which has few nutrients. Always remember, the greener the vegetable, the more chlorophyll and nutrients. Iceberg lettuce is provided at McDonald's, Burger King and other fast food franchises. When they provide a salad in coach, it is iceberg, but in first class they serve wild greens, romaine, or spinach.

In contrast, in low-income communities, the variety and quality of produce is tragic. I have seen some low-income stores where they only had three live items in the store—apples, oranges, and onions. You then go to an upscale affluent suburban food store and there could literally be one hundred types of fruits and vegetables.

60 Minutes did an expose of the French population to ascertain why they have less heart disease than Americans. Satan would have us believe it is because they consume a glass of wine after dinner. What is often not mentioned is that the French spend a lot more time than Americans purchasing food and there is a greater abundance of produce. The American lifestyle at lunchtime is to go to the fastest restaurant. Ideally, we don't even leave our cars, we drive through and in ninety seconds or less, we have our lunch and ninety seconds later, we've eaten. In contrast, the French spend time at lunch and in the evening shopping at the produce market for food. Their lunch could not be confined to thirty minutes. Their produce has fewer pesticides and is sprayed with copper. There are over two billion pounds of pesticides sprayed on American crops and over 3,000 chemicals added to processed food. I would suggest that you never eat produce that you have not sprayed and washed with pesticide remover.

The American lifestyle values speed and shopping in bulk. Did you ever wonder why government cheese and peanut butter never spoil? How could it? It was dead from the onset. For many of us, the objective is to go to these large discount stores and buy food for the month, if not several months. The American approach is "stock up and eat out." We have large freezers and cabinets and we store large quantities of canned and frozen goods, and meats.

Satan laughs, and God cries. God wants us to choose life. Food that you purchased weeks and months ago has very little life. There are very few minerals and vitamins. We exacerbate the problem when we cook these items that were already dead. You see, before we cooked them, they had very few nutrients. When cooked, oxygen and enzymes are lost. Ninety-three percent of the nutrients are destroyed by cooking and 84 percent by freezing. Our bodies can not live without oxygen and enzymes.

This book will not be easy for some because it is more than about food and diet. Ultimately, it is about lifestyle. It is about choosing life in an environment geared towards death. It is almost as challenging being a Christian trying to live holy in a decadent society.

I am begging and pleading with you that daily you eat from this day forward, something real. Your body is alive, and in order to remain alive and energetic, it must have real food. *Giving a live body dead food is the major reason for health problems.*

There was a weekly study done on a sample population of students who consumed only 4.7 servings of fruit. Many of the students consumed no fruit at all. Another study showed for many youth, the only vegetable that they consumed were potatoes in the form of french fries and potato chips. Another study of 11,658 adults indicated 41 percent did not consume any fruits.[1] This decision to consume more raw food will force you to shop more frequently. Is your health important enough to you that you are willing to shop for produce two or three times a week? Isn't it amazing how live food does not last long? It forces you to shop frequently.

To illustrate the life giving properties of raw food, try this experiment. Secure three carrots and cut off half of all three. Boil one, bake one, and then place each carrot in a pot of soil. Only the raw carrot will produce growth. It has the same effect in our bodies. One of the best-known studies of raw versus cooked foods with animals was a 10-year-research project conducted by Dr. Francis M. Pottenger, using 900 cats. Dr. Pottenger fed all 900 cats the same food, with the only difference being that one group received it raw, while the others received it cooked. The results dramatically revealed the advantages of raw foods over a cooked diet. Cats that were fed raw, living food produced healthy kittens year after year with no ill health or premature deaths. But cats fed the same food, only cooked, developed heart disease, cancer, kidney and thyroid disease, pneumonia, paralysis, loss of teeth, arthritis, birthing difficulties, diminished sexual interest, diarrhea, irritability, liver problems and osteoporosis (the same diseases common in our human cooked-food culture). The first generation of kittens from cats that were fed cooked food were sick and abnormal, the second generation were often born diseased or dead, and by the third generation, the mothers were sterile.

The following is an account of an interesting three-part experiment comparing the effects of raw foods versus cooked foods with rats. It has been found that a group of rats were fed diets of raw vegetables, fruits, nuts and whole grains from birth grew into completely healthy specimens and never suffered from any disease. They were never ill. They grew rapidly, but never became fat, mated with enthusiasm and had healthy offspring. They were always gently affectionate and playful and lived in perfect harmony with each other. Upon reaching an old age, equivalent to 80 years in humans, these rats were put to death and autopsied. At that advanced age their organs, glands, tissues and all body processes appeared to be in perfect condition without any sign of aging or deterioration.

A companion group of rats were fed a diet comparable to that of the average American and included white bread, cooked foods, meats, milk, salt, soft drinks, candies, cakes, vitamins and other supplements, medicines for their ailments, etc. During their lifetime these rats became fat and, from the earliest age, contracted most of the diseases of modern American society including colds, fever, pneumonia, poor vision, cataracts, heart disease, arthritis, cancer and many more.

Most of this group died prematurely but during their lifetime most of them were vicious, snarling beasts, fighting with one another, stealing one another's food and attempting to kill each other. They had to be kept apart to prevent total destruction of the entire group. Their offspring were all sick and exhibited the same general characteristics as the parents.

As this group of rats died one by one or in epidemics or various diseases, autopsies were performed revealing extensive degenerative conditions in every part of their bodies. All organs, glands and tissues were affected as were the skin, hair, blood and nervous system. They were all truly total physical and nervous wrecks. The same conditions existed in the few which survived the full duration of the experiments.

A third companion group of rats was fed the same diet as the second group to an age equivalent to about 40 years in humans. They displayed the same general symptoms of the second group—being sick and vicious so that they had to be separated to prevent them from killing each other and stealing one another's food.

At the end of this initial period all rats in this group were placed on a strict fast, with only water to drink for a period of several days. Then they received the natural (raw) diet of the first group of rats. This diet was alternated with periods of fasting and within one month the behavioral pattern had changed completely so that the now docile, affectionate, playful creatures were once again able to live together in a harmonious society and from this point on **never suffered any illness**.

Several rats were put to death and autopsied at the end of the initial period revealing the same general deterioration as that exhibited in the second group of rats. However, the remaining rats lived out the full duration of the experiment, to the equivalent of 80 years in humans, and when they were autopsied there were no signs of aging or deterioration or disease—just as those in the first group. The obvious disease, degeneration, and deterioration of body parts evident in their first half of life had been completely reversed and excellent health restored.[2]

The same principles apply to human life. Our cells cannot regenerate without live food. Raw food has oxygen while cooked food has carbon dioxide. It reminds me of the Israelites in the desert where God provided them with fresh manna daily. Satan's food can remain on the shelf forever. It is already dead, the problem is we continue to consume it.

Eating correctly is challenging for adults. It is even more challenging for children. When you send your child to a party and would like for your child to eat nutritious food and the only food offered is pizza, hot dogs, hamburgers, cake and ice cream, it becomes very challenging to parents. Children like many adults are greatly affected by peer pressure and have a tremendous desire to be part of the group. It is very difficult finding an American party with carrot sticks, orange wedges, apples, bananas, and salad. It is even more challenging when they become adolescents and start dating. It is difficult trying to find live food during the daytime. It is like trying to find a needle in a haystack. Finding live food at night is also difficult, especially in low-income communities.

Business people plan meetings around food. Banquets dictate food. Holidays, food, and weight gain all seem related. When you think of summer, barbecue comes to mind. What does a nutrition conscious person do when the menu consists of barbecue ribs, chicken, potato salad, iceberg lettuce, white bread, and beer?

I mentioned in the chapter on Satan, that if there was an immediate negative reaction after consuming ribs or beer most of us would change. I have discovered many people do receive a negative reaction, but the pharmaceutical industry comes to the rescue and advertises don't worry about what you ate, just take this particular drug afterwards and the pain will disappear.

That's the American lifestyle. Let me contrast the American lifestyle with other countries. Have you ever heard the term "third world"? Anyone thinking would realize there must be a first and a second. I've often wondered what makes America first? Oh, first in heart disease, cancer, diabetes, and strokes. There are countries that do not have our level of income, but have a much higher level of health. The people who live the longest, who have been able to cash-in on God's promise of 120 years, are the Vilcambas, (Ecuador), Himalayans, (northern India), Abkhazians, (Soviet Union) and Hunzas (Pakistan).[3] These groups are primarily vegetarians, poor, and have very little health care.

We may have the richest country in the world and the most expensive health care, but it does not mean we are healthy. When you compare our health to Asia, American men have a 26 time greater chance of prostate cancer than Chinese men. Japan has far less incidence of heart disease and cancer than Americans.[4]

Let me describe what happens to Americans very early in life. From infancy to age two, we give our children cow's milk. In the following chapter, *You Are What You Eat*, more will be said about this. We also give children canned food filled with salt and sugar. This is the way we start our children. From age two to 18 our children are allowed to eat everything and not required to eat green food. I understand why most people would not want to be vegetarians. When you ask people what they are having for dinner, they respond only with meat. You wonder if they mean that literally, does that mean they are only having steak? No, what it really means is that is what they value most. In addition, they will have a carbohydrate, and overboiled tasteless vegetables. Another reason why most people would not want to become vegetarians is all the spices, creativity, and effort allocated to preparing the meat could also have been invested in preparing the vegetables.

From infancy to early adulthood, because we are fearfully and wonderfully made, it looks as if we are still healthy. Children are energetic while eating anything and everything and not gaining weight, even though research indicates more children are becoming obese. Seventy percent of obese two-year-olds will be obese adults. Forty-one percent of obese seven-year-olds unfortunately will be obese adults. Ten percent of children, twenty percent of adolescents and thirty percent of adults are obese due to the American diet.[5] But all things considered, many Americans pimp God's grace and believe they can consume whatever they want without consequences. Our childhood lifestyle stays with us for the rest of our lives. If we have not been taught in childhood to value drinking water and eat live food there is a very good chance it will never be valued. Many young adults continue to eat fast food with little exercise.

Weight begins to increase and our health decreases. From age 35–50 health problems become significant. We become more dependent on drugs and doctors to address the problem. We still don't get it. We don't realize that you are what you eat and what you don't eliminate. Your body is alive and in order for it to remain alive it needs live food. Many die at 50, but others at that age accept their poor health and become totally dependent on doctors and drugs. For some reason doctors and drugs are inseparable. More will be said about this in subsequent chapters.

Let me describe the typical American day. We fasted during the night while sleeping. We awake and break the fast (breakfast). You don't break a fast with a heavy meal unless you don't know any better. Since many of us do not, we break our fast with bacon, sausage, eggs, biscuits, grits, coffee, cigarettes, and "cereal with our sugar." For lunch, we have a 70 plus fat gram sandwich. I'm sure you're aware of the fat grams in a Big Mac and other fast food sandwiches, especially with cheese, french fries, and a shake. For dinner, we have steak or fried chicken, white rice, which has very little nutrients, and overcooked, dead mixed vegetables. We snacked throughout the day with Snickers, pop, and potato chips. We conclude the evening with ice cream and cookies.

Many Americans have tried to reduce their fat gram intake, but their calories increased. How long do you think you can live off that diet? What kind of health and energy does that diet offer? When you compare that diet to our grandparents' not only did they consume more fruit and vegetables, but much of their meat was used to season beans and greens. You've heard the commercial, "you've come a long way baby." It's advertised for cigarettes. The same thing can be said for many of us as we've come a long way financially and now consume meat at every meal.

My wife and I often tease each other. We make a very good income and yet are excited about having a pot of beans or greens. Beans have no cholesterol, are rich in iron, high in fiber, low in fat, and high in protein, vitamin B, calcium, and potassium. We make enough money to eat steak, but choose life. The issue is not money, the issue is life. The Himalayans, Hunzas, Vilcambas, and Abkhasians have little money, but excellent health.

I've also observed that not only was the move from rural to urban dramatic, but from a warm to a cold climate. Have you ever noticed in the summertime you don't have as much desire to eat heavy food as you do during the winter? During the summertime, many are satisfied with a piece of watermelon, cantaloupe, or salad. It's difficult when it's five below zero to get excited about a salad versus a hot bowl of sausage gumbo. It becomes more challenging in a cold, urban environment to eat right. When you live in a cold, urban environment, it encourages people to stock up for the month. But God wants us to choose life regardless of temperature and locale.

How many times do you exercise per week? For many of us our last exercise class was our mandatory high school gym class. Yet we want to compare ourselves to our grandparents who exercised daily. Living in an urban environment and working in the information age has created a sedentary lifestyle.

In contrast, when we were farmers without cars, we walked to work and school. This was exercise. In our current lifestyle, we have to create artificial conditions for exercise. People walk around the park, or on their treadmills. Their walking is not necessary; it is for exercise. Many of us ride bikes going nowhere! We ride a stationary bike while in years past we rode a bike to and from work and school, but some exercise is better than none at all. Have you ever bought a piece of exercise equipment that you rarely use? Have you ever purchased membership at a health club that you seldom take advantage of? Why is it that many of us do not exercise? How is it that the President of the United States can find time to exercise with his demanding schedule and many of us cannot?

I was very disappointed when the late mayor Harold Washington died in office. Do you know how hard it was to elect an African American mayor in one of the most racist cities in the country? Why did Harold Washington gain 90 pounds in six years of office? Can you imagine African

Americans lost City Hall because of Harold Washington's diet and lack of exercise? Why didn't he realize that if he was going to work an eighteen-hour day, seven days a week that his body deserved the best diet and exercise? You would think that if you are going to demand that much from your body, you would give your body plenty of water, fruit, salad, exercise, and vitamins in order to function at maximum capacity.

I have found that as much as I enjoy exercise, it's even more enjoyable to find something that you like. I know that many of us have a tendency to stop exercising not only because of our lifestyle and time constraints, but many of us have not found something that we enjoy. What type of exercise do you enjoy? What types of game do you like playing? If you can find a marriage between what you enjoy and exercise you are very successful.

I truly enjoy running, swimming, and tennis. Exercising is no longer a chore, it's something I enjoy. I feel like a child all over again. On my birthday, I take the day off and act like a child. I wake up in the morning, have my devotion, and praise my Lord and Savior for another year. I run three laps, one for the Father, one for the Son, and one for the Holy Spirit. I swim and then go to the batting cage to see if I can still hit like when I was thirteen. I go bowling, and cap off the day playing tennis with my wife. I have been blessed with a godly wife who can play tennis for hours!

Find something that you enjoy and use time management skills. If you are waiting for the appropriate time to exercise, seldom will it happen. You need to assign a time to the exercise. You need to make exercise important. I'm very impressed with my sister, who is a single parent, and has a very demanding career. She knows evenings will be filled with dinner and homework, so she exercises three days a week during her lunch hour, at the health club.

There is no excuse for not exercising. We can start by walking up the stairs. Research shows that 90 percent of Americans agree that exercise is important, but only 15 percent actually exercise on a regular basis, and 76 percent fail to exercise at all. We spend almost 40 billion dollars annually on equipment, but unfortunately most of it collects dust. Exercise reduces heart attacks by 64 percent.[6] Exercise is also great for relieving stress. Exercise is easier in the summer. Try playing golf, tennis, running, or swimming in the wintertime. Exercise is essential for the elderly, especially females who have a greater chance of osteoporosis and fractures. Exercise can prevent injuries. These activities would require additional income. Not all Americans can afford these exercises. Lack of income is still no excuse for not exercising. We can run in place at home. We can do sit ups and push ups at home. Everyone has a floor.

We must spend more time outdoors including winters. Americans spend 90 percent of their time indoors. Some spend almost the entire winter indoors. Indoor air is 90 times more polluted than outdoors.[7] Our bodies can survive 40 days without food, four days without water, but less than four minutes without oxygen. Many of us have bodies starving for fresh air. We must each day go outdoors and slowly take in deep breaths of oxygen.

Many Americans after age thirty have sedentary lifestyles and cannot walk a block. We are becoming an obese and lazy nation. Almost one-third of Americans are obese and close to 50 percent of African American women over 40. Yankee stadium removed 9000 seats, because the size of American population had widened and people were complaining that the seats were too small.

It is unfortunate how Satan works. Many Americans like hearing stories about some health and exercise guru who had a heart attack. The first thing you'll hear is "That's why I don't exercise, I don't want to get a heart attack." Unfortunately, many of us actually look for these stories to rationalize our sedentary lifestyle. I know being a vegetarian since 1973, exercising regularly, and writing this book, that some people will be pleased if I "catch a cold," become ill, or suffer from a disease. They will then negate everything I've written in this book because of what happened to me.

Many Americans are not aware that many marathon runners, and professional ball players, including one who passed recently, suffered from a selenium deficiency which contributed to the heart attack. It had nothing to do with the exercise. If anything exercise made him stronger, but exercise alone cannot negate nutritional deficiencies. We must consciously take vitamins and minerals due to a loss in topsoil. Vitamin E is one of the essential vitamins that we need to consume. If you want to take the minimum requirement of 15 iu it would require consuming 248 slices of wheat bread, 16 dozen eggs, and 20 lbs. of bacon. We must take vitamins!

LIFESTYLE

1900	2000
Breast milk	Cow's milk and powdered milk
Walked three miles to school and work	Bus or car to school and work
Worked in the field	Sit at a desk
Absorbed more sun	Absorb light from electricity

LIFESTYLE AND HABITS

Sweated daily	76 percent never exercise or sweat
Breathe clean air	Inhale pollutants
Drank mineral water	Drink less water and more polluted
Consumed an abundance of fruits and vegetables	Consume less than four pieces of fruit and vegetables per week
Consumed greens and beans regularly and pot liquor from the greens	Consume little greens or beans
Consumed meat primarily to season the food	Consume meat at every meal
Consumed four pounds of sugar annually	Consume 155 pounds of sugar annually
Very few snacks	Snack constantly
Consumed complex carbohydrates full of fiber	Consume refined carbohydrates with little to no fiber
Obesity was not a factor	One-third obese
The soil had 103 minerals and vitamins	The soil has very few minerals
Told stories	Watch television
60 percent attended church and prayer was in school	Less than 40 percent attend church and guns are in school

One of 33 died of cancer	1 of 3 die of cancer
Three thousand died of heart disease	Two million die annually
Ten percent divorced	50 percent divorce

While I am very concerned about longevity, I am more concerned about the quality of your health. The media speaks a great deal about cancer, and heart disease, but I think the greatest problem is fatigue. It is not normal to be fatigued. I am not saying an 80-year-old will have the same energy as an eight-year-old, but I believe the major reason for fatigue is not due to age, but the food we eat.

In the following chapter, we will show the correlation between food and health.

YOU ARE WHAT YOU EAT

Most of us have heard the phrase, "You are what you eat." Do you live to eat or do you eat to live? Do you read the labels on the food you eat? One simple rule of thumb is that if you can't pronounce it you should not eat it or if you can't pronounce it you should research it before you consume it. Wouldn't it be great if you can eat whatever you wanted and there would be no consequences to your health? Many of us do eat whatever we want, unfortunately there are consequences.

As mentioned in an earlier chapter, because the consequences are not immediate, many of us feel we can continue to eat whatever we want. With the pharmaceutical industry, there will always be a pill to address the problem.

The average American annually consumes 155 pounds of sugar, 55 pounds of fat, 300 sodas, 20 pounds of candy, 63 dozen donuts, 50 pounds of cake, cookies and pies, 20 gallons of ice cream, and 12 pounds of potato chips. Forty-eight percent of Americans utilize fast food franchises for at least one meal daily.[1]

The four major addictions are sugar, caffeine, nicotine, and alcohol. One of the major problems with fast food is oxidized fat, which is terrible for the arteries. Have you ever tried to reheat fast food french fries? French fries cut from a potato and fried, can be reheated. French fries from a frozen bag have been dead for so long Jesus could not resurrect them!

Pepsi and Coca-Cola are excellent for cleaning automobile battery cables. The acid content is ideal for removing residue from cables. They are terrible for your liver,

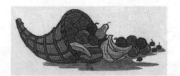
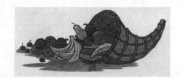

kidneys, and pancreas. If you visit a supermarket you will witness numerous aisles, but only one for produce. The profit margin is very small in this aisle due to spoilage. The greatest profit margin is in aisles where food never spoils.

The food industry can make far more profit selling potato chips than selling potatoes. Food manufacturers release 12,000 new products annually. Most stores reserve an entire aisle for potato chips, popcorn, pretzels, corn curls, and other combinations. What percentage of your food budget is allocated for produce? How much time do you spend in the produce aisles?

When I first became health conscious in 1973, I was taught the concept of the six whites.

The Six Whites (man made)	Natural (God made)
White rice	Brown rice
White flour	Wheat flour
White bread	Wheat or rye bread
White salt	Himalayan Crystal Salt, Spike, Sea salt
White sugar	Unrefined honey or molasses
White noodles	Wheat noodles

I would like you to compare a piece of white bread to 100 percent wheat bread. Feel the difference and squeeze the

the white bread. If you moisten the white bread it feels like white paste. That gluey substance clogs our bloodstream, arteries, and veins. White flour products have lost 75 percent of their selenium. This trace mineral reduces your risk of heart disease and cancer. I would suggest consuming whole wheat products and taking this vital supplement through vitamins. In order to increase shelf life of wheat products, food manufacturers remove the vital substance – wheat germ. White bread has no fiber and Satan tells us white bread is enriched. We think the garden of Eden story is ancient, but just as Satan deceived Eve, he's still deceiving us. God's bread is still the best. Have you noticed that God gave us wheat bread, brown rice, wheat flour, sea salt and honey in their 100 percent natural state?

How can you take out what the Lord put in, add chemicals, and call it enriched? White rice is inferior to God's brown rice. White flour is inferior to God's wheat flour. White refined sugar is inferior to unrefined honey and molasses. I am often asked, "What can I eat?" People need alternatives. The alternatives to the six whites are superior.

Table salt increases our blood pressure. Satan is so deceptive, that we don't realize 70 percent of the salt we consume was added by food manufacturers or chefs. Many of us were addicted to salt before we picked up the salt shaker to add our 30 percent.

The seventh white is milk. This is a food for infants. Milk is not to be consumed for the rest of your life. God in his infinite wisdom gave every mother milk designed for her child. Do you see cows giving their calves human milk? Do you see dogs giving their puppies cat milk? Do cats give their kittens dog milk? Are these animals smarter than humans? Is this another ploy from Satan?

Satan and his cohorts can not make money off breast milk, therefore they encourage humans to use cows for milk, which profits the dairy association. Unfortunately, since 1930 little girls have started their menstrual cycle six months earlier for every decade. Young girls are now starting their menstrual cycle as early as eight years of age. The reason for this is the protein increase in the diet. When I speak in high schools, it's hard to distinguish students from teachers. Cow's milk develops the body; breast milk develops the brain. Cow's milk has 300 percent more protein than human milk. The following charts illustrate that cow and breast milk are not identical.

HUMAN	COW
Casein percentage 50%	82%
Whey percentage 60%	18%
Calcium-Phosphoric Ratio 2 to 1	1.2 to 1
Vitamin A per liter 1898	1028
Niacin per liter 1470	940
Vitamin C per liter 43	11
Reaction in the body Alkaline	Acidic[2]

COMPARISON OF THE MILKS OF DIFFERENT SPECIES

	Mean values for protein content per cent.	Time required to double birth weight (days)
HUMAN	1·2	180
MARE	2·4	60
COW	3·3	47
GOAT	4·1	19
DOG	7·1	8
CAT	9·5	7
RAT	11·8	4·5

If you thought the paste from adding a little water to white bread was significant, the amount of casein in cow's milk is literally destructive. Casein is a substance that is used to make glue. I believe this is the major contributor to fibrosis. If women would eliminate dairy products, they could shrink their fibroids.

Can you imagine the effect of glue inside the bloodstream, arteries, veins, and organs? Almost 40 percent of children less than six years of age have chronic ear infections. This is a result of consuming cow's milk. If you or your children are suffering from a cold, which is an excess amount of mucus in the body, one of the most effective ways to rid the body of the mucus is to eliminate the consumption of cow's milk. Many humans, specifically African Americans, do not have the enzyme lactase to digest cow's milk. Milk is toxic and mucous forming.

While this book is about health, I like to mention that not only is human milk the ideal milk for infants, but the bonding between mother and child is indescribable. It illustrates the unconditional love and nurturance God has for us.

We live in a culture where Satan has made the breast a sexual object and not what God intended –the organ to transmit food to His children. We now have some mothers more concerned about society frowning about them breast feeding their children. Ironically, while a large percentage of White mothers have begun to breast feed their children, in "third world" countries, mothers who were breast feeding their children, were called savages and began to imitate the West and are using cow's milk or Nestles' bottled formula. This has caused major health problems never experienced before.

The alternative to cow's milk would first be breast milk, followed by soy, coconut, or sesame seed. Soy is an amazing food. It comes from the soybean, which possesses genistein, an excellent anti-oxidant (an anti-oxidant is a chemical that destroys free radicals which daily attack the immune system). It also has a protease inhibitor which is ideal for cancer prevention. There are many products which are derivatives of the soybean including soy margarine, cheese, and ice cream. Tofu also comes from soybeans.

I would like for you to read the labels on ice cream. It is unbelievable the number of chemicals within ice cream. It is one of the most detrimental foods available. Maybe that's why Americans enjoy it so much. It seems the less food in a product and the more chemicals the more we enjoy it.

Another very popular item in the American diet is black pepper. How many times do you use black pepper daily? For many of us we have food with our pepper. Black pepper irritates the stomach lining. The alternative to black pepper is cayenne pepper. It is a blood cleanser, strengthens the heart, and regulates blood pressure.

I've met many people over the years who have told me they are eating better and are consuming more salads. I often go out with these people for lunch or dinner and they take me to their favorite salad bars. They know that since I'm a vegetarian I would love a salad bar. When we sit down to eat, I notice they have a plate full of salad, but very little lettuce, tomatoes, cucumbers, broccoli, and other vegetables. Satan has done it again; he has taken over the salad bar. People think they are consuming a salad when it's really shrimp, chicken, potato, and macaroni salad. Can you imagine a salad filled with meat and carbohydrates and no vegetables? In addition, it is covered with salad dressing, cheese, croutons, and bacon bits.

The problem is compounded at many salad bars by using iceberg lettuce. All lettuce is not the same. Iceberg lettuce has little to no nutrients and is cheaper than other lettuce. I have appealed to many restaurants to change, but most don't because of price and consumers don't demand a better lettuce, which is the foundation of a salad. The greener the vegetable the more life it possesses. A wonder food that God wants all to have is chlorophyll. It has a similar structure to the human hemoglobin molecule. Chlorophyll is ideal for circulatory concerns, digestion, respiratory, and builds the immune system.

When I'm in my hotel room after a speaking engagement, I order a salad. Sometimes, I forget to be thorough with waiters. I must first make sure they give me romaine, red leaf, green leaf, or spinach. I then tell them no bacon bits. Why do they put pork on salads?

Unfortunately, people are attempting to lose weight by eating a salad, but use a salad dressing with 17 grams of fat. This also occurs with a baked potato, where we use so much salt, pepper, butter, cheese, and sour cream that we cannot see the potato. Did we really want the potato or the condiments?

One of the major objectives I have in this book is for you to realize that you are God's child, fearfully and wonderfully made, and God wants you to prosper in all things, including your health. I want you also to realize that unfortunately because the topsoil has eroded the minerals it becomes your responsibility to secure them. Each day we must consciously secure these 103 minerals and vitamins. *You cannot be sick if you have an adequate amount of those 103 nutrients.* To achieve this goal will require more than simply taking an inadequate multivitamin. It will require a good diet and specific vitamins.

YOU ARE WHAT YOU EAT

Some of the Major Vitamins, Minerals, and Nutrients

Source	Food	ODA (Optimal Daily Allowance)	Significance
Vitamin A	Carrots	5000 iu	eye sight
Vitamin B1 Thiamin	Brewer's Yeast	5mg	cell development
Vitamin B2 Riboflavin	Total Cereal	5mg	energy
Vitamin B3 Niacin	Product 19 Cereal	20mg	skin protection
Vitamin B12 Cobalamin	Clams	400mcg	prevents anemia
Vitamin C	Acerola	500mg	builds immune system
Vitamin D	Cod Liver Oil	400 iu	bone density
Vitamin E	Wheat Germ	400 iu	delays aging
Vitamin K	Beans	120mcg	prevents blood clotting
Calcium	Milk	1500mg	bone density
Iron	Clams	15mg	blood enhancer
Magnesium	Pumpkin Seeds	500mg	cell development
Selenium	Haddock	200mcg	reduces heart disease
Zinc	Oysters	20mg	cell growth

Only nine percent of Americans eat five servings of fruits and vegetables on a daily basis. Fifty percent of Americans consume no fruit and vegetables on any given day. They did not make a distinction between raw or cooked. My position is that when we advocate five servings of fruits and vegetables it should not include fruit cocktail, apple pie, peach cobbler, banana pudding, frozen or canned vegetables, or french fries.

The above have very few enzymes. An entire chapter could have been devoted to enzymes. They enable us to digest food and absorb it into our blood. I encourage you whenever you eat cooked food to take enzymes. One of the major reasons why many of us are fatigued and have this middle age feeling is due to the lack of enzymes in our food. If you have a desire to increase your energy level do one of two things, either eat more raw food and/or take enzymes with cooked food.

Have you ever had a headache? I have been blessed when I became a vegetarian in 1973 to never have a headache. There are foods that contribute to headaches. These foods include caffeine, chocolate, cheese, processed meats, alcohol, MSG, and Nutrasweet. Do you consume any of these foods? Before you take your next aspirin, and most Americans are dependent and addicted to aspirin, consider changing your diet. If you eliminate the foods mentioned earlier and drink more water your headache disappears. One of the main reasons we have headaches is because our blood is toxic and void of nutrients. If we increased our chlorophyll and enzymes, we would experience less headaches. If we inhaled more outdoor air, practiced deep breathing, and exercised it would reduce our headaches.

I will give you a list of foods that will give you life. Foods are not the same. There are superior foods. There are foods that will give you energy. Some foods delay the aging process. Aging is a result of free radicals that attack our bodies. Your body needs anti-oxidants to fight these free radicals. Foods with vitamins C, E and beta carotene are equipped to fight these free radicals and delay the aging process. If you would like to live longer, become more energetic, and look well take note to the following foods: almonds, broccoli, carrots, kelp, figs, flax oil, omega 3 oil, grapefruit, wheatgrass, soy products, honey, garlic and green vegetables which include, kale or any other type of greens, red leaf, green leaf, romaine or endive lettuce, and spinach.

These are just some of the wonder foods. My desire is that on a daily basis you consume these foods, all the fruit that you can imagine, and eight glasses of water. If you then want to eat some other foods you enjoy then that would be your compromise. It is not my desire to make your life and diet boring. My desire is to try to provide alternatives that will improve your health.

The one thing I will not compromise is that your body is made of 103 minerals and vitamins and in order for you to sustain your body, you need to be more scientific about the food you eat. You cannot achieve this going to Burger King for breakfast, McDonalds for lunch and Wendy for dinner. You must take control of your health, it does not belong to fast food chains, pharmaceutical companies, and doctors.

Let's return to those wonder foods and elaborate on what they do for your body.

Almonds	Rich in fiber, vitamin E and selenium. They also provide good fat.
Broccoli	An antioxidant, it has large amounts of calcium. It removes excess estrogen, and provides a great source of fiber.
Carrots	Excellent source of beta carotene, it is a anti-cancer agent, it boosts our immune system, protects our arteries, and improves our vision.
Kelp	It kills viruses, restores and rebuilds our immune system. It detoxifies the body and nourishes the thyroid gland.

Grapefruit	Decreases our cholesterol level and our chances for atherosclerosis. It builds our immune system and burns fat.
Greens	They have antioxidants and cancer fighting agents. They are filled with beta carotene and chlorophyll.
Wheatgrass	It is considered the complete food with 92 of the 103 vitamins and minerals that our bodies require. It has 17 amino acids. Wheatgrass is a body cleanser, body builder, and possesses liquid oxygen. Liquid is preferred, but also available in tablet form. Fifteen pounds of wheat grass is the nutritional equivalent of 350 pounds of vegetables.
Soybeans	It provides hormone balance, is an anti-cancer agent, and decreases our cholesterol. It possesses the valuable nutrient genistein, which reduces estrogen production.
Unrefined honey	Contains 18 of the 22 amino acids.
Garlic	It decreases our blood pressure. It avoids blood clotting and decreases the chance of heart disease and cancer.
Flax oil and omega 3 oil	Excellent sources of HDL and decreases the chance of heart disease and cancer.

Fats are not all the same. There are basically four types of fat: saturated, polyunsaturated, monounsaturated, and transfat. Saturated and transfat cause our arteries to harden. They are filled with LDL (bad) cholesterol. Polyunsaturated and monounsaturated fat are high HDL (good) cholesterol. These fats decrease our chances of having a heart attack. Flax oil and Omega 3 oil are also essential for building up our HDL.

Other super foods to add to your diet are spirulina, blue-green algae, royal jelly, noni, bee pollen, barley grass, and chlorella.

One of the greatest decisions I ever made was consuming food through juicing. Have you ever visited a health food store and had a cup of carrot juice? Did you notice how many carrots were required to produce a 16 ounce cup of carrot juice? Did you notice the carrots are larger? Not only will juicing your food allow you to consume a greater amount than the desired five daily servings of fruit and vegetables, but the body can use it instantly because it requires no digestion. *There is no greater gift that you can give your body than fresh vegetable juice on a daily basis.* Notice I did not mention fruit juices. It is not that I'm against orange juice, or other combinations of fruit. I have noticed that what Satan did to most salad bars he is trying to do to juice bars.

Many juice bars over the years are providing less vegetable juice and more fruit juices and smoothies. The latter is what Americans want while the former is what Americans need. Many juices bar owners tell me they discontinued vegetable juices because of low demand. Wheatgrass is considered the complete food. It has more minerals, vitamins, and amino acids than any other food. You literally have to be a detective to find a juice bar that juices wheatgrass. It is no comparison to vegetable juices, and vegetable juices are no comparison to fruit juices. Remember Satan comes to kill and God came to give life. The next time you visit a juice bar—choose life. Do you love yourself enough to either buy a juicer and juice daily or visit a juice bar daily?

There is no more demanding process on the body than digestion. Many people after a meal are tired. If you think exercise is demanding, it is a pale comparison to the amount of work required by your liver, intestines, and pancreas for digestion.

Unfortunately, less than two percent of the American population avoids coffee and caffeinated tea. One cup of coffee takes 24 hours to pass through your kidneys. It is only a matter of time that we move from coffee and pop to the dialysis machine. Caffeine is only added to soda to make it addictive; it is not necessary for taste. Unfortunately, most Americans start their day with either coffee or caffeinated tea. Wouldn't it be great if we started our day with fruit or vegetable juice? It would be fantastic if we started it off with wheatgrass!

There is a rumor in America that many of us are starving on a full stomach. Can you imagine that? We eat everything, but the food is void of minerals and vitamins. Only one American per 1000 escapes malnutrition in the richest country in the world. There are other ethnic groups in "third world" countries who are not suffering from malnutrition. Their diet is full of chlorophyll and enzymes.

In the following chapter on elimination, we will look beyond what you eat, to what you did not eliminate.

YOU ARE WHAT YOU DON'T ELIMINATE

The greatest threat to the American population is constipation. I know this is supposed to be a health book, but I would like to review some basic math problems.

How many meals and snacks do you have on a daily basis? How many bowel movements do you have on a daily basis? If your first answer is greater than your second answer, then my next question is where is the food?

The rule of thumb is if you eat three times a day you should eliminate three times a day. In America the medical definition of constipation is less than two bowel movements per week, which in my opinion is unacceptable. Even with that criteria, there are 30 million Americans who are constipated and 80 million Americans have irritable bowel syndrome. One third of the American population suffers from hemorrhoids. Americans spend over $500 million on laxatives.[1] The average American adult passes 80 to 120 grams of stool daily. The average adult in Africa, India, and the Pacific Islands passes 300 to 500 grams daily.[2] Have you ever kept garbage in your house for a week during the summer without air conditioning? How would the garbage smell? What would it look like? Did it look different on the first day and the seventh day? That describes what happens in our bodies. Our body temperature is 98.6 degrees and if we consumed a meal on Monday and seven days later a portion remains it has fermented, petrified, become toxic, and contaminated our blood supply and vital organs.

The next question is where does it go if it is not eliminated? It reminds me of a sewer system. Have you ever had

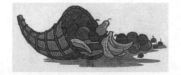
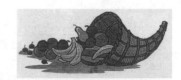

a toilet or kitchen sink backup? In our bodies, food that backs up begins to damage the gallbladder, pancreas, kidney, liver, and the heart. It clogs the arteries and forms cakes of waste along the small and large intestinal wall and the colon, which contributes to irritable bowel syndrome, hemorrhoids, and chrones disease. I believe you are what you do not eliminate.

The medical profession does not examine the colon until they believe there is a risk of colon cancer. Chiropractors, naturopaths, herbalists, and colon therapists believe the colon is the best indicator of health. Does your doctor? Do you know the state of your colon? Do you know how much waste is there? How long has it been there? What do you plan to do to eliminate the waste?

Did you know that when an autopsy was performed on John Wayne that the weight from the waste in his colon exceeded 40 pounds? I do not believe he was the exception to the rule. We could lose weight and improve our health if we eliminated what we ate. Why does the medical profession accept two bowel movements per week?[3] Ideally, we should eliminate what we have consumed in less than twelve hours. Why is it taking so long for Americans to eliminate their food? Why is colon cancer second only to lung cancer and yet the easiest to detect? Why are young people including super athletes like Darryl Strawberry and Eric Davis, becoming victims to colon cancer?

In the previous chapter, we mentioned the importance of consuming live food that possesses enzymes, which are important for nutrient absorption and elimination. One of the major reasons why Americans are suffering is because we have moved from a predominantly raw diet to predominantly cooked food diet. We have moved from live food to dead food. If you look at Americans in the early 1900s, they consumed more raw food that possessed the 103 nutrients from adequate topsoil. A century later, Americans consume very little raw food or nutrients.

I don't know if it's because we are becoming lazy or it's part of the culture, but many people shy away from raw food because it requires more chewing. We can aid in the elimination process if we not only consume more raw food, but if we chewed our food better. Ideally we should chew thirty times before swallowing.[4] Many Americans eat food so overcooked it has the texture of baby food. Could the problem be that 155 pounds of sugar has rotted our teeth and we try to avoid chewing?

One of the major reasons why we are having a problem with elimination is that we are consuming food void of fiber. There is no fiber in meat, eggs, or dairy products. In the previous chapter, we mentioned the six whites which have little to no fiber. If you compare the amount of fiber in white bread, flour, rice, and noodles to 100 percent wheat, rye, or brown products you would have a better appreciation of what happens in your small and large intestines and colon. The fiber becomes a brush to remove waste from the intestinal and colon walls. You can eliminate constipation with fiber. Fruits and vegetables are full of fiber. Wouldn't it be cheaper and less painful if we simply ate fiber than to suffer and spend money on constipation, hemorrhoids, irritable bowl syndrome, and chrone's disease?

FIBER CONTENT
OF COMMON FOODS

FOOD ITEM	FIBER (g/kg)	FOOD ITEM	FIBER (g/kg)
Blueberries	15.2	Ground Beef	0
Brussels Sprouts	13.5	Sirloin Steak	0
Oat Flakes	13.5	Lamb Chops	0
Pumpkin	12.0	Pork Chops	0
Cooked Carrot	9.6	Chicken	0
Brown Rice	8.1	Ocean Perch	0
Swiss Chard	6.8	Salmon	0
Lettuce	6.3	Cheddar Cheese	0
Cucumber	5.7	Whole Milk	0
Applesauce	5.3	Eggs	0

Source: *Nutritional Almanac* (Revised), Nutritional Research, Inc.,
John D. Kirshman, McGraw Hill Book Co., New York, 1979

5

In an earlier chapter on the body, we mentioned that you could have a bachelors, masters, or doctorate degree and not understand the function of your colon. The same applies for food combining. Most people have not been taught that there is a science for how food should be combined. Our bodies work to perfection like cars when they are properly maintained. Our digestive system works better if we separate solids from liquids. Historically we did that. People did not drink while eating watermelon, cantaloupe, honeydew melon, oranges and grapefruits. As our diets began to change and we ate more cooked food, filled with chemicals, and void of nutrients, we felt a need to "wash it down" because there was very little water in the food. It has now become the norm to eat and drink simultaneously. The problem is our digestive system becomes confused. There are different enzymes needed to digest liquids and solids. The body literally goes on strike and neither are digested properly. When the body finally makes a decision to digest one or the other, it chooses the liquid. This further delays the digestion of solid food.

My request is that you try not drinking while eating. The rule of thumb is to either drink 30 minutes prior to the meal or 90 minutes after the meal, but every effort should be made to separate the two. Another important food combination rule is the separation of fruit with any other food. Fruit after liquid is the easiest to digest, but if it is in the stomach with any other food then it will ferment and you lose its nutrients. Watermelon, honeydew, and cantaloupe are even more demanding. They should be consumed separately. Try to avoid combining these fruits in a fruit salad.

I often have problems on airplanes and restaurants. They are trying to do better by offering fruit, but they offer fruit for dessert, which negates the fruit combining rule. Fruit should be the appetizer not dessert! Many times, I will ask the flight attendant what is for dessert? If they say fruit, I will ask if I can have my dessert first. They look at me strangely, but my body appreciates the effort. The third food combining rule is the separation of raw and cooked food. The salad should be consumed before cooked food.

The fourth rule of food combining is the separation of proteins and carbohydrates. This has been a major challenge for me over the years because I love sandwiches and potato chips. Earlier, I mentioned we can not allow food to control us. I felt convicted and throughout the writing of this book, I have denied myself potato chips.

The typical American diet is hamburger and french fries. It tastes great, but the body cannot digest it properly. We have to die to the flesh and live to the spirit. We have to ask ourselves do we live to eat or do we eat to live? We have to ask ourselves what is more important? Hamburger and fries that will stay in the body for extra hours or days or separating the two and having it eliminated in less time.

The beauty of this option, is that it does not negate that you can still consume carbohydrates and protein. I'm not taking away your hamburger or French fries (even though they are both fried with few enzymes), you will still be able to consume them, but separately. You can have a hamburger and vegetables at one meal and french fries and vegetables at another. In the hierarchy of food digestion, liquids, water fruits, other fruits, salad, cooked vegetables, carbohydrates, and proteins.

Notice, protein, in this case meat, is last on the list. Our bodies have the greatest challenge digesting meat. If you look at the intestinal and colon track of lions, tigers, and humans they are not the same. For animals that consume meat, the intestinal and colon track is less than one foot long. Those animals eat it raw and within hours it is eliminated. Our bodies are not designed like lions and tigers. Our small and large intestine are 30 feet long, and when you add our colon you have a very long intricate system. I mentioned 30 feet long, obviously we are not 30 feet tall, so the 30 feet of small and large intestine is a very complex woven intricate system with many curves. The challenge is for our digested food to make it through 30 feet of intestinal curves.

On average it takes 10 to 14 days for pork to be eliminated from the system. It takes beef 8 to 12 days, chicken takes 4 to 8 days, and fish takes 3 to 5 days. There is still a portion of the meat that will remain indefinitely. Many meat eaters have chosen to eliminate red meat for fish and chicken. This was a very good move, because it eliminated worms and uric acid. Unfortunately, fish and chicken will only reduce cholesterol by five percent and are also void of fiber. In comparison, raw fruits and vegetables take six hours. You do the math, and ask yourself do I really want to put that kind of pressure on my system?

My suggestion is rather than spending 500 million dollars on laxatives, consume more fruit, fiber, dates, raisins, figs, and granola. I would also recommend juice therapy. Some of the excellent juices which are effective in accelerating the elimination process are wheatgrass, celery, spinach, carrot, and beet. You can add apple juice as a sweetener. There has become an increasing number of colon cleansers on the market. While I am in favor of these laxatives, I am concerned with over reliance on herbal cleansers. I have had people tell me they can now eat whatever they want because they have an herbal cleanser that will remove what they ate.

Satan is at it again. The objective is to realize that we are fearfully and wonderfully made and not to think that you can eat "chitlins" and take an herbal cleanser to alleviate the problem. Please don't think that an herbal cleanser can remove all the waste from the colon, small intestine, large intestine, liver, kidneys, and your blood stream. Herbal cleansers are an aid, not meant to replace a diet of live food. There are some excellent herbal cleansers, which include psyllium, casara sagrada, flax seed, beans, oat bran, and apple pectin. My wife and I have achieved excellent results with one-half cup each of apple juice and water, two tablespoons each of liquid chlorophyll and hydrated bentonite, and one tablespoon of physillium. This has been commercially packaged by Nature Sunshine and is available at our office African American Images (773) 445-0322.

Another strategy to improve elimination is an enema. Everyone should know how to give themselves an enema. Mothers could avoid emergency room visits if they gave their babies an enema to reduce their temperature. Enemas can be an excellent resource to improve your overall health. When you know you have eaten something wrong, feeling sluggish, experiencing stomach irritation, before taking another laxative or drug, consider giving yourself an enema. The traditional enema I am referring to would be with water. Another enema would be a coffee enema. Caffeine is excellent to clean battery cables and your colon. Janet Jackson raves about her success with coffee enemas. Warm water enemas should be used to eliminate waste, cool water enemas are ideal to eliminate gas, and cold water enemas tone the colon. If you have a disease, add wheatgrass to your enema. The results are amazing!

Enemas have their origin in Egypt, thousands of years ago. African doctors understood the importance of keeping the colon clean. Just as many of us are illiterate about enemas, we seem to be equally confused about colonics. This in my opinion, is a higher form of an enema. There are health practitioners called colon therapists who use colonics to improve our health. I would encourage all readers to give your body one of its greatest experiences—a colonic. While I appreciate enemas, I have to do all of the work. What I like most about the colonics, is that I simply go into the colon therapist's office, lay on a table, meditate while the colon therapist is sending water through my colon and intestines. The colon therapist alters the water temperature between cool and warm, letting water in and waste out. Over a period of 30 minutes, 5 to 15 gallons of water have circulated through the colon area.

What is amazing is that you could fast for 21 days and take either an enema or colonic daily and there would still be waste being eliminated. It shows the magnitude of waste. After a colonic, I feel almost "born again." You feel like you have a new lease on life. You promise yourself that you will be more careful with what you eat, because you realize how involved it is to remove waste. Unfortunately, for many the promise does not last long.

The medical profession used to give colonics, but unfortunately in the 1940s they discontinued the practice. They decided colonics were time consuming taking 45 minutes and it was more cost efficient if they prescribed laxatives. Forty-four percent of the American population suffers from heartburn, indigestion, and constipation. They think the solution lies in the drug store.

It is one thing for doctors to have made a decision to discontinue colonics, but the American Medical Association (AMA) has in many states made it unlawful for anyone to provide colonics. I can't fault someone for being illiterate about colonics if they live in a state where it is not legal. I encourage you to ascertain whether colonics are legal in your state. If unavailable, visit another state and appeal to your local AMA to make them available.

The last suggestion I have on improving elimination is fasting. There are numerous references in the Bible about fasting.

The major attribute for fasting is to have a closer walk with God. Fasting not only has a spiritual benefit, but also physical. The body works better when we consume less food, spread our meals over a greater period of time, and eliminate snacks. Many Americans eat from sun up to sundown. Our digestive system never has a chance to rest.

My first suggestion would be if we must consume three meals, let's make sure they are spread out as far apart as possible. The first meal, breakfast, should be lighter, preferably fruit and juice. The second suggestion would be two meals a day. There are numerous types of fasts. There are some people that define a fast as simply the elimination of a particular type of food. A person may decide to avoid eating meat or sweets for a particular period of time. Others define a fast as the Daniel fast, which is described in the Bible as only consuming fruits and vegetables. Fasting also varies based on the time frame. Some people define a fast as sun up to sundown. My concern about that fast is that some people negate the benefit by waking up before the sun and eating as much as they can and repeating the mistake at sundown. Other fasts would be a juice fast where you only consume liquids. The last fast would be only the consumption of water. This is the most demanding fast.

Because our bodies are fearfully and wonderfully made, our bodies can fast on water for more than 40 days. Our bodies are 80 percent water and this fast gives our body what it needs the most. The body is intelligent; it will feed off of itself, while eliminating waste material. This is excellent for cell regeneration.

In conclusion, we must become more concerned about elimination. This reflects the state of our health. In the following chapter, we will discuss the very controversial debate between protein and carbohydrate advocates.

70

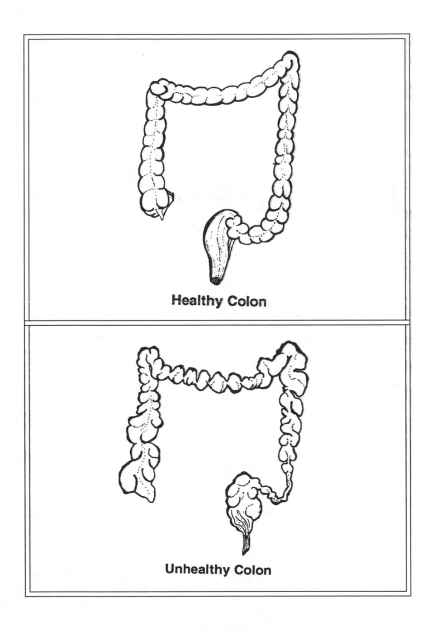

Healthy Colon

Unhealthy Colon

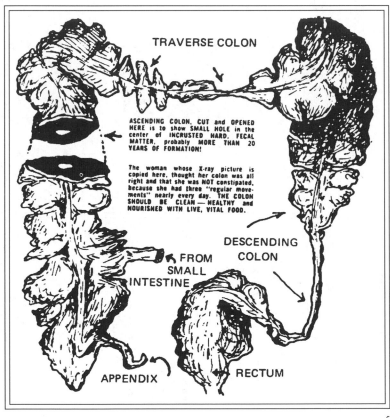

TRAVERSE COLON

ASCENDING COLON, CUT and OPENED HERE is to show SMALL HOLE in the center of INCRUSTED HARD, FECAL MATTER, probably MORE THAN 20 YEARS OF FORMATION!

The woman whose X-ray picture is copied here, thought her colon was all right and that she was NOT constipated, because she had three "regular movements" nearly every day. THE COLON SHOULD BE CLEAN — HEALTHY and NOURISHED WITH LIVE, VITAL FOOD.

FROM SMALL INTESTINE

DESCENDING COLON

APPENDIX

RECTUM

5

THE BIG DEBATE:
PROTEINS VS. CARBOHYDRATES

One of the things that I enjoy most about writing is the amount of research that is required. If a student or writer is honest, they have an open mind as they pursue their research and are willing to make changes. I mentioned I am a vegetarian, therefore obviously I have a bias toward eating meat, but there is research encouraging us to consume more meat.

Historically, research has shown the major contributor to heart disease, cancer, strokes, and high blood pressure is a high fat diet. In 1988, research was introduced that the major contributor to heart disease, diabetes, and obesity is a low fat diet filled with refined carbohydrates.[1] There have been many best selling books by these protein advocates that have captured the attention of the American public. These authors include Dr. Atkins, Drs. Michael and Mary Eades, Dr. Steward, Barry Sears, and others.

One of the most frequent questions I am asked as a vegetarian is where do I get my protein? It's interesting that adults ask this question based on their limited information they received as children in elementary schools from curricula, sponsored by the pork, beef, and dairy associations. I wonder why people don't ask me and themselves where do they get their calcium, phosphorus, potassium, iron and all the other 103 minerals and vitamins that we all need? I wonder if the same people that ask me the protein question also ask themselves how much protein do they get after cooking? I also wonder if the people asking me that question ever thought where do cows, gorillas, elephants, horses, and rhinoceros and other vegetarian animals secure their protein?

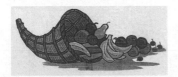
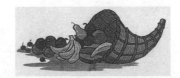

73

If you observe cows they get their protein from grass. All food has protein which consists of 22 amino acids. The body produces 14 of these essential amino acids, the remaining eight come from our diet. Earlier, I mentioned wheatgrass is a complete food, because it has all eight essential amino acids. There are numerous green foods that possess a large number of those eight essential amino acids. Another ideal source is beans. It is true that meat is an ideal source for these eight amino acids if eaten raw. When cooked, it becomes an incomplete food void of many of the eight essential amino acids.

Let me give some perspective on how much meat Americans consume over a 72 year life span. The average American will consume 11 cattle, 3 lambs, 310 pigs, 45 turkeys, 1100 chickens, and 862 pounds of fish without enzymes. In an earlier chapter, we discussed the loss of topsoil. One major reason is livestock. It requires 3.25 acres to feed every meat eater. It requires one-sixth of an acre to feed a vegetarian. Eighty percent of our corn and 95 percent of our oats are consumed by livestock. That quantity of grain could feed the entire world! One acre of land will provide 40,000 pounds of potatoes or 250 pounds of beans.[2]

PERCENTAGE OF CALORIES
FROM PROTEIN

LEGUMES

Soybean sprouts	54%
Mungbean sprouts	43%
Soybean curd (tofu)	43%
Soy flour	35%
Soybeans	35%
Soy sauce	33%
Broad beans	32%
Lentils	29%
Split peas	28%
Kidney beans	26%
Navy beans	26%
Lima beans	26%
Garbanzo beans	23%

VEGETABLES

Spinach	49%
New Zealand spinach	47%
Watercress	46%
Kale	45%
Broccoli	45%
Brussels sprouts	44%
Turnip greens	43%
Collards	43%
Cauliflower	40%
Mustard greens	39%
Mushrooms	38%
Chinese cabbage	34%
Parsley	34%
Lettuce	34%
Green peas	30%
Zucchini	28%
Green beans	26%
Cucumbers	24%
Dandelion greens	24%
Green pepper	22%
Artichokes	22%
Cabbage	22%
Celery	21%
Eggplant	21%
Tomatoes	18%
Onions	16%
Beets	15%
Pumpkin	12%
Potatoes	11%
Yams	8%
Sweet potatoes	6%

GRAINS

Wheat germ	31%
Rye	20%
Wheat, hard red	17%
Wild rice	16%
Buckwheat	15%
Oatmeal	15%
Rye	14%
Millet	12%
Barley	11%
Brown Rice	8%

FRUITS

Lemons	16%
Honeydew melon	10%
Cantaloupe	9%
Strawberry	8%
Orange	8%
Blackberry	8%
Cherry	8%
Apricot	8%
Grape	8%
Watermelon	8%
Tangerine	7%
Papaya	6%
Peach	6%
Pear	5%
Banana	5%
Grapefruit	5%
Pineapple	3%
Apple	1%

NUTS AND SEEDS

Pumpkin seeds	21%
Peanuts	18%
Sunflower seeds	17%
Walnuts, black	13%
Sesame seeds	13%
Almonds	12%
Cashews	12%
Filberts	8%

Data obtained from "Nutritive Value of American Foods in Common Units," U.S.D.A. Agriculture Handbook No. 456

3

ESSENTIAL AMINO ACIDS OF SELECTED FOODS

(grams per day) AMINO ACIDS	Rose's Minimum Requirem.	Rose's Recom. Requirem.	Corn	Brown rice	Oatmeal flakes	Wheat flour	White beans	Potatoes	Sweet Potatoes	Taro	Asparagus	Broccoli	Tomatoes	Pumpkin	Beef club steak	Egg	Milk
Tryptophan	.25	.50	.66	.71	1.4	1.4	1.8	.8	.8	1.0	3.9	3.8	1.4	1.5	3.1	3.8	2.3
Phenylalanine*	.28	.56	6.13	3.1	5.8	5.9	10.9	3.6	2.5	3.0	10.2	12.2	4.3	3.0	11.2	13.9	7.7
Leucine	1.10	2.20	12.0	5.5	8.1	8.0	17.0	4.1	2.6	5.2	14.6	16.5	6.1	6.0	22.4	21.0	15.9
Isoleucine	.7	1.4	4.1	3.0	5.6	5.2	11.3	3.6	2.2	3.0	11.9	12.8	4.4	4.3	14.3	15.7	10.3
Lysine	.8	1.6	4.1	2.5	4.0	3.2	14.7	4.4	2.1	3.4	15.5	14.8	6.3	5.5	23.9	15.3	12.5
Valine	.8	1.6	6.8	4.5	6.4	5.5	12.1	4.4	3.4	3.5	16.0	17.3	4.2	4.3	15.1	17.7	11.7
Methionine*	.11	.22	2.1	1.1	1.6	1.8	2.0	1.0	.4	.6	5.0	5.1	1.1	1.0	6.8	7.4	3.9
Threonine	.5	1.0	4.5	2.5	3.6	3.5	8.5	3.4	2.1	2.7	9.9	12.5	4.9	2.7	12.1	12.0	7.4
Total protein	20	37 (WHO)	109	64	108	120	198	82	45	58	330	338	150	115	276	238	160

One pound of meat requires animals to consume 2500 gallons of water. On a daily basis to feed the average meat eater will require 4,000 gallons of water in contrast to 300 gallons to feed the average vegetarian. More than 50 percent of the American water supply is consumed by livestock.

Fifty-five percent of all antibiotics are fed to animals. Seventy percent of all pesticides are used for meat and dairy products.[4] DDT, MSG, and nitrates are added to most meats. Ninety-nine percent of meat eaters have a significant level of DDT. The meat industry is very much aware that if it does not add these chemicals to the meat, it would turn brown or gray. If your children are diagnosed with attention-deficit-disorder, I would encourage you to eliminate these pesticides along with sugar.

When animals are killed their urine remains. One pound of meat generates 18 grams of uric acid, while our liver and kidneys only excrete eight grams daily. Can you imagine retaining 10 grams of uric acid on a daily basis over a 72 year life span? Unfortunately, because uric acid cannot be totally eliminated from the body, it crystallizes in our joints creating arthritis and rheumatism. Americans think that arthritis and rheumatism are a natural result of aging, when in reality arthritis and rheumatism are an unfortunate reality from meat consumption.

In an earlier chapter on the body, we mentioned one of the functions of the liver is to filter toxins from our body. That is also the function for all animals. We should not consume livers from other animals, because it is filled with toxins. While the liver is an excellent source of iron, there are cleaner sources.

Throughout this book, we have mentioned that more Americans have become obese. The figure is greater for those who are overweight. Historically, Americans have been told to reduce their fat consumption and eat more carbohydrates. Unfortunately, the number of people overweight and obese has risen, even with a low-fat diet. This triggered the debate between protein and carbohydrate advocates.

The most popular American foods are white bread, white rolls, crackers, donuts, cookies, cake, and alcohol.[5] The American diet is 46 percent carbohydrates, 43 percent fat, and 11 percent protein. Interwoven in this debate between proteins and carbohydrates has been the relationship between highly refined carbohydrates, which are filled with sugar, and the impact it has had on Type II diabetes.

Only ten percent of the American diabetes population is Type I. These victims were born with the disease. They do not produce an adequate amount of insulin and must rely on injections. The remaining 90 percent of the American diabetic population is not genetically driven, but directed by their over consumption of refined sugar-filled carbohydrates.[6]

In earlier chapters, we mentioned the American population has gone from four pounds of sugar annually to almost 155 pounds. God's body was not designed to consume that much sugar. If you went to a supermarket and asked the manager to remove all products with sugar the store would eliminate 90 percent of its inventory. I would love to see a sugarless store.

What are the consequences of consuming 155 pounds of sugar? The pancreas has to produce insulin to balance the glucose level which rises with sugar consumption. The pancreas overreacts and produces excess insulin. The consequence of excess insulin is hyperinsulinemia. You cannot separate diabetes from high blood pressure, strokes, heart disease, obesity, and cancer.

Before 1988, the assumption was that proteins and fat were increasing the cholesterol level, high blood pressure, strokes, cancer, heart disease and obesity. For that reason nutritionists and doctors recommended a low fat, low protein diet. The accepted assumption was a decrease in protein and in fat would reduce heart disease, cholesterol, high blood pressure, and strokes. The medical experts did not think the culprit was sugar.

Who would have thought that sugar could have a significant effect on heart disease, cholesterol, cancer, high blood pressure, and strokes? Excess insulin stores fat and is a major reason for weight gain. The American population is consuming less fat, but more calories and sugar. Insulin stores excess fat and starts the production of cholesterol, which contributes to high blood pressure, cancer, strokes, and heart disease.

There is also a relationship between excess sugar consumption and cancer. Cancer feeds off glucose. In a subsequent chapter on healing, we will discuss this in detail. Suffice to say at this point we could reduce cancer if we simply reduced, or ideally eliminated, sugar from our diet. Excess insulin makes the kidneys retain more fluid, which leads to high blood pressure and swelling. The alternative hormone to glucose is glucagon. The benefits of glucagon which results from consuming protein and fat is that it burns fat. It releases fat from cells and fluids from the kidneys.

If the major objective is to lose weight, Americans have been very disappointed with the low fat, high carb diet. I'm in total agreement with Drs. Atkins, Eades, Steward, Barry Sears, and other proponents that say refined carbohydrates filled with sugar not only increase weight, but also contribute to major diseases. A high refined carbohydrate diet contributes to weight gain because people continue to eat because although they are full they remain malnourished.

From a vegetarian perspective, I see nothing wrong with the consumption of fruits. If you read some of the above authors carefully, they suggest that fruit also contributes to diabetes and excess insulin production. I totally agree but there is no benefit from the consumption of ice cream, cake, cookies, and the bulk of the American diet.

Consuming more meat is acceptable and palatable to most Americans who want a quick fix with little to no exercise and no real sacrifice in the diet. The trade off is no ice cream, cake, and cookies for all the meat, eggs, and cheese your heart desires. For many Americans who love proteins this was not a sacrifice. To those who love both, it is simply giving up one for the other with the benefit of losing weight. You can imagine the pork, beef, chicken, seafood, and dairy associations have loved this diet. In addition, it has created a great degree of controversy since most people like showing the experts they were wrong advocating a low fat, low protein diet.

There has been much discussion about the consumption of eggs. If you like eggs, regardless of research, you will probably continue to consume them and find research to support your position. Please carefully read the sponsor of the research. Many favorable reports on eggs have been sponsored by the egg industry. The American Heart Association (AHA) recommends a maximum of four eggs per week. If you are against animal by-products or believe past research that espouses eggs increase cholesterol, you will avoid their consumption. Eating eggs is a major contributor to allergies along with milk.

I believe the protein advocates are correct. Dietary cholesterol is different from cholesterol produced by the body. There is also a difference between HDL (good) and LDL (bad) cholesterol. Egg consumption slightly increases LDL but significantly increases HDL.

In defense of the AHA, egg consumers should reduce if not eliminate consumption if they have a high LDL reading which results from consuming saturated fat and they should eliminate saturated fat (meat) if they eat eggs. I would further suggest avoiding eggs if your cholesterol level is greater than 160 and blood pressure exceeds 120/80. The ideal cholesterol level is 150. It is almost impossible to have heart disease at this level. The median cholesterol level for

Americans is 210. Do you know your cholesterol and blood pressure level? You should know before you eat another egg. In the following chapter on vegetarianism, I will show other ways to secure protein and avoid any risk of LDL and arteriosclerosis.

Let's review to make sure we are clear on the intricacies of protein, carbohydrates, sugar, cancer, high blood pressure, heart disease, stroke, diabetes, and obesity. When we consume refined carbohydrates there is a tremendous increase in our glucose level. A candy bar could increase our glucose level by 50 points. The pancreas responds and produces insulin to decrease the glucose level. For many of us, this happens numerous times throughout the day.

Have you ever wondered why children can consume so many sugar-filled products and gain less weight than adults? The answer is they have a higher metabolism, greater exercise, and God protects them from hyperinsulinemia. God is so awesome that when his children first come into the world He knows their bodies cannot handle a large amount of insulin because children's cells are extremely sensitive to insulin. The body provides a smaller amount of insulin to reduce the blood sugar level.

The problem is that over a period of time the body has less sensitivity to the amount of insulin being produced and as we become older the pancreas produces an excess amount. How unfortunate, most people are consuming the same if not less sugar as adults, but the body is less sensitive to excess insulin production. Diabetes has now become a major health hazard in America not due to "nature" (Type I 10 percent) but due to "nurture" (Type II 90 percent). The American diet of excess sugar created the diabetic dilemma.

I'm sure someone is wondering, there has to be a drug to correct the problem. The answer is no. There is no drug or pill that can correct this problem. This will require you to be disciplined and reduce and/or eliminate sugar and refined carbohydrates from your diet. Please remember diabetes is interwoven with high blood pressure, high cholesterol, obesity, stroke, heart disease, and cancer.

There is a direct relationship between obesity and high blood pressure. There are 35 million Americans in this country who are obese and 40 million Americans who have high blood pressure. Among the obese, hypertension is three times more common than among the non-obese. High tryglyceride levels are twice as common among the obese than among the non-obese. If we decreased our consumption of refined carbohydrates that would reduce the amount of insulin produced. A decrease in insulin production decreases the amount of fat being stored and cholesterol produced. A decrease in obesity will contribute to a reduction in blood pressure. A reduction in the production of cholesterol also reduces blood pressure. The above will reduce our chances of strokes, heart disease, and cancer. Obesity, which is excess body fat, makes estrogen, which contributes to breast cancer.

Let's look at several groups around the world and the affect proteins and carbohydrates have had on their health. There has been much discussion about the French population and while they have a similar diet to Americans, they have less incidence of heart disease. Many people felt it was the glass of wine. I mentioned earlier, they consume more fruits and vegetables. The major reason for the difference lies in sugar consumption. Americans consume 155 pounds of sugar while the French only consume 26 pounds.[7] This is very close to what Americans consumed in the 1900s when diabetes, heart disease, cancer, and obesity were non-existent.

Another group I think would be very interesting to observe would be the Eskimos. They consume very few carbohydrates and none during the winter season, and yet not only live a long life, but have very little incidence of heart disease, diabetes, high blood pressure, and obesity. There was a study done on the Aborigines in Australia, who did not possess Type II diabetes until they were "civilized" with the American diet. There was a tremendous increase in Type II diabetes and the subsequent illnesses.[8]

There was a study done by a surgeon, Captain Cleave, who wrote the classic book, *The Saccharine Disease.* He documents that as awesome as God's body is designed, after 20 years of a bad diet, it begins to decline. He looked at several populations exposed to the American diet. He looked at Eskimos of North America, the Masia of East Africa, and the people of Yugoslavia and Poland. What he observed among all four groups before there was a change in diet was no incidence of diabetes and resulting diseases. Unfortunately, after they were exposed to sugar, there was a tremendous incidence of these diseases.[9]

I totally agree with the high protein advocates about the elimination of sugar and refined carbohydrates. They have done us all well by documenting the relationship between sugar, diabetes, hyperinsulinemia, obesity, high blood pressure, strokes, heart disease, and cancer.

The average American diet consists of 46 percent carbohydrates, 43 percent fat, and 11 percent protein. The protein diet advocates recommend between 30 and 50 percent protein and 30 to 50 percent fat and the remainder complex carbohydrates.

83

If you read them carefully, some recommend ten percent or less carbohydrates. Some have even recommended the complete elimination of carbohydrates.

My first concern to the protein advocates is will their diet provide them with all 103 minerals? My second concern is that while there is weight reduction with an increasing consumption of protein and decreasing refined carbohydrates, much of that loss is water. Carbohydrates contain water, and our bodies are 80 percent water. A diet that reduces water consumption in its food can put the body in ketosis, and the body becomes dehydrated. Ketosis reflects a body that is highly acidic and filled with ketones. These are toxic substances that the body is trying to eliminate. The body is losing water trying to dilute ketones.

Protein advocates acknowledge their diet creates bad breath and body odor. Have you ever wondered why this diet creates bad breath and body odor? They are signals of a clogged colon. Why does this diet create a clogged colon? Because there is less water in the colon, more toxic waste, and no fiber, which is necessary for proper elimination.

If you listen carefully to these protein advocates they don't recommend this diet for the duration. Why not? Oprah Winfrey has stated numerous times – diets do not work. It requires a change in lifestyle. A high protein diet loses water, but it cannot be continued without the body experiencing ketosis. The high protein diet does not provide you with the 103 minerals and vitamins. Dr. Atkins is wise to take 36 supplements not just because of topsoil erosion, but because of the limitations in his diet.

A high protein diet causes a tremendous amount of work for the kidneys, liver, and colon. The amount of uric acid and toxic waste in meat can literally destroy the kidneys, liver, and colon. A high protein diet is the major reason that heart disease and cancer are the leading American killers. The following charts illustrate this concern.

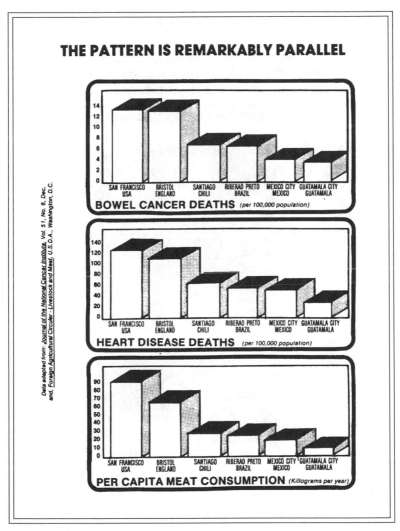

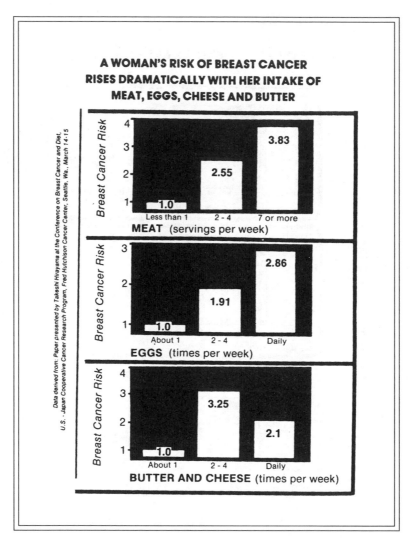

A WOMAN'S RISK OF BREAST CANCER
RISES DRAMATICALLY WITH HER INTAKE OF
MEAT, EGGS, CHEESE AND BUTTER

11

86

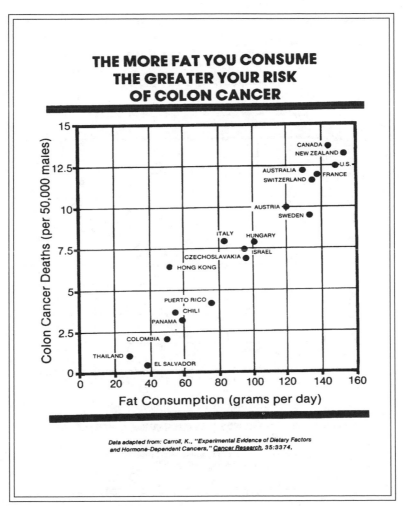

THE MORE FAT YOU CONSUME THE GREATER YOUR RISK OF COLON CANCER

Data adapted from: Carroll, K., "Experimental Evidence of Dietary Factors and Hormone-Dependent Cancers," *Cancer Research*, 35:3374.

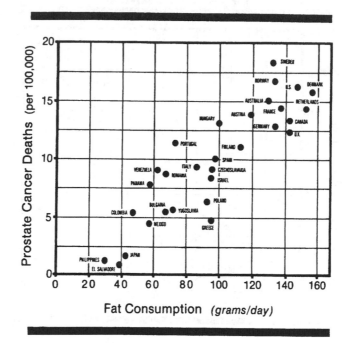

AGAIN & AGAIN
THE SAME PATTERN

Data adapted from: Reddy, B.S., et al, "Nutrition and Its Relationship To Cancer," *Advances in Cancer Research*, 32:237,

13

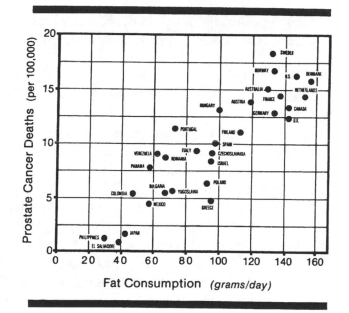

**AGAIN & AGAIN
THE SAME PATTERN**

Data adapted from: Reddy, B.S., et al, "Nutrition and Its Relationship To Cancer,"
Advances in Cancer Research, 32:237,

14

Secondly, our bodies have to have a balance between acid and alkaline. The pH range is between 0 and 14, with 1 to 7 being acidic and 8 to 14 being alkaline. The ideal is 11 or 80 percent alkaline. Sixty million American meat eaters suffer heartburn due to its acidity. The solution is not taking an antacid, but eating more fruits and vegetables which have an alkaline effect on the body. Disease flourishes in an acidic body. A body that is highly acidic not only creates bad breath and body odor, but causes damage to kidneys, liver, and constipates the colon. Animal fat at 98 degrees hardens, clogs the arteries, and contributes to high blood pressure and heart disease.

A diet that is highly acidic requires the body to create balance. The body has no other choice but to take calcium from its bones. This is the major reason for osteoporosis. The question that I have to these protein advocates is how can a country that has the greatest milk consumption have the greatest incidence of osteoporosis? You've seen commercials and billboards with Spike Lee, Whoopi Goldberg, Patrick Ewing and others sponsored by the Dairy Association encouraging greater milk consumption. Osteoporosis is a major problem for the elderly. Satan has tricked us again. Many of us were unaware that we were robbing our bodies of calcium by consuming more meat.

Forty-five percent of 65-year-old women in America suffer from osteoporosis. Male vegetarians had an average measurable bone loss of only 3 percent. Male meat eaters had an average measurable bone loss of 7 percent. Female vegetarians had an average measurable bone loss of 18 percent, and female meat eaters had an average measurable bone loss of 35 percent.[15]

IS OSTEOPOROSIS
DUE TO CALCIUM DEFICIENCY
OR EXCESS PROTEIN?

STUDY No.	CALCIUM INTAKE -milligrams-	CHANGE IN CALCIUM BALANCE WITH A LOW-PROTEIN DIET	CHANGE IN CALCIUM BALANCE WITH A HIGH-PROTEIN DIET
1	500	+31	-120
2	500	+24	-116
3	800	+12	-85
4	1400	+10	-84
5	1400	+20	-65
AVERAGE	920	+19	-94

Study No. 1 . . . Anad, C., "Effect of Protein Intake on Calcium Balance of Young Men Given 500 Mg Calcium Daily," *Journal of Nutrition*, 104:695, 1974

Study No. 2 . . . Hegsted, M., "Urinary Calcium and Calcium Balance in Young Men as Affected by Level of Protein and Phosphorous Intake," *Journal of Nutrition*, 111:53, 1981

Study No. 3 . . . Walker, R., "Calcium Retnetion in the Adult Human Male As Affected By Protein Intake," *Journal of Nutrition*, 102:1297, 1972

Study No. 4 . . . Johnson, N., "Effect of Level of Protein Intake   rinary and Fecal Calcium and Calcium Retention of Young Adult Males," *Journal of Nutrition*, 100:1425, 1970

Study No. 5 . . . Linkswiler, H., "Calcium Retention of Young Adult Males As Affected by Level of Protein and of Calcium Intake," *Trans New York Academy of Science*, 36:333, 1974

Data as per McDougall, Dr. John, *McDougall's Medicine*, New Century Publishers, New York, 1985

FACTOR	HUMAN	COW
Casein percentage	50%	82%
Whey percentage	60%	18%
Calcium-Phosphoric	Ratio 2 to 1	Ratio 1.2 to 1
Vitamin A per liter	1898mg.	1028 mg.
Niacin per liter	1470mg.	940mg.
Vitamin C per liter	43mg.	11mg.
Reaction in the body:	Alkaline	Acidic

COMPARISON OF THE MILKS OF DIFFERENT SPECIES

	Mean values for protein content per cent.	Time required to double birth weight (days)
HUMAN	1·2	180
MARE	2·4	60
COW	3·3	47
GOAT	4·1	19
DOG	7·1	8
CAT	9·5	7
RAT	11·8	4·5

We mentioned the Eskimos earlier and their heavy protein diet with less incidence of heart disease, cancer, and diabetes. The unfortunate reality is that Eskimos have the highest rate of osteoporosis in the world. The Bantus in a "third world" country consume much less calcium than Americans and yet have one of the lowest incidence of osteoporosis in the world.[17] Americans consume 70 percent of their proteins from animals. The Chinese consume seven percent from animals. The American diet only consists of 11 grams of fiber daily. The Chinese consume 77 grams of fiber daily. The Chinese have very little incidence of osteoporosis.[18]

I pray that this chapter has not been too confusing. There were many issues discussed which could have been an entire book. In summary, we need to reduce or eliminate sugar and refined carbohydrates from our diet. The taxation on our bodies because of refined carbohydrates causes diabetes and stimulates excess production of insulin. Hyperinsulinemia causes obesity, high blood pressure, strokes, heart disease, and cancer.

While it is our desire for everyone to reach their natural weight we need to change our lifestyle not just our diets. How unfortunate that the debate has been reduced to the lesser of two evils: sugar or meat. The former makes you obese along with other problems and meat destroys your kidneys, liver, and colon while giving osteoporosis. Both contribute to heart disease and cancer.

God wants you to choose life. There are other options than sugar and protein, diabetes and colon cancer. The following chapter on vegetarianism provides a healthy lifestyle.

VEGETARIANISM

People would much rather see a sermon than hear one. When we talk about our Lord and Savior Jesus Christ to an unbeliever, it is one thing to quote scripture, but it is far more significant for them to see how your relationship with the Lord has made a difference in your life. The same applies to diet. It is one thing for me to write a book about diet, but I think it's more significant if I share with you a little about my experience and what my vegetarian diet has done for me.

I have been a vegetarian for almost 30 years. I have never missed a day of work. I am very energetic. I attribute this to God's grace, diet, and exercise. If you want to feel better and become more energetic—try it! I was a junior in college in 1973, and had the typical American diet. I did not read the labels on the food that I ate. I consumed everything and the most important criterion was taste. My roommate had just read a book on vegetarianism and he shared it with me. I'm the kind of person that if I hear or read something, and it's logical, I have the ability to move beyond theory to practice and to implement this new body of knowledge. Earlier that day, before reading the book I had bacon for breakfast, a salami sandwich for lunch, and pork chops for dinner. As I read this book, I became fascinated. There were numerous ideas I had never thought about. The chart below describes some of these revelations.

Parts of the body	Carnivorous	Human
Teeth	Incisors are undeveloped molars are very long sharp and pointed	Incisors are well developed molars for crushing and grinding
Jaw	Up and down motion for tearing or biting	Equipped for grinding motion

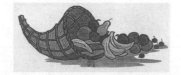
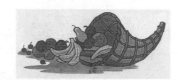

95

Saliva	Acid saliva geared to digestion of animal protein lacks ptyalin, a chemical which digests carbohydrates	Alkaline saliva adopted to the digestion of carbohydrates
Stomach	Simple round sack, which secretes 10 times more hydrochloric acid than humans	Oblong in shape complicated in structure
Intestine	Three times the length of the trunk	12 times the length of the trunk
Colon	Short and smooth designed for prompt evacuation not digestion	Long and involved nutrients are digested then evacuation
Liver	Eliminates a large amount of uric acid	Retains large amount of uric acid
Hands	Claws for tearing flesh	Fingers adopted to pluck fruits and vegetables and killing
Urine	Acidic odor	Alkaline

I had never been exposed to this information. It seemed so logical. I looked at my hands and it was obvious that I could not kill an animal on the spot with them or my mouth. It became clear to me that animals who eat meat, kill it and eat it instantly. For humans who eat meat the length of time involved between when the animal is killed and when they eat it, could exceed six months. If the meat packing plant did not provide the tremendous amount of chemicals to the meat no human regardless of how much they love meat would consume it. Many of us still possess the naive view of meat processing that we were taught in primary grades. We were never told this curriculum was paid for by the meat packing association. The following describes what most of us believe.

VEGETARIANISM

At last the special day has come,
She is so very proud,
As she looks down at her very
  first egg
She clucks and clucks so loud.

It is usually only a few days after she is in the laying house that she lays her first egg. Chickens do actually 'cluck' or 'sing' after laying an egg . . . it really seems to make them happy. Incidently, there are no roosters (male birds) in these laying houses. The hen just lays eggs naturally The rooster is required for a fertile or hatching egg.

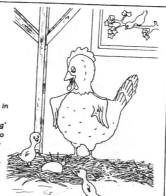

The cow now goes with many others
To the pasture to drink water
  and eat grass.
Some may stop at the salt box
To take a lick of salt as they pass.

In the summer the cows are turned out to pasture to eat grass. The dairy farmer keeps a salt box in the pasture because cows need salt. Cows also need a lot of water. It is important in helping them to digest food and to make milk. Water also helps to keep the cow cool in the summer. She may drink as much as twenty gallons of water a day.

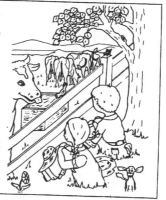

1

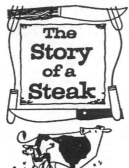

The Story of a Steak

Before you have a steak (whether it's porterhouse or chopped), a cow has to have a calf. This is the story of one particular calf.

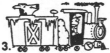

1. This calf was born on a Texas ranch. Several acres of grazing land are required to support each cow and calf.

2. As a yearling, the calf was sold to an Iowa farmer for "finishing" in feed lot. Proper feeding of corn and protein supplements adds many extra pounds and a lot of extra eating quality to our beef.

3. After several months in the feed lot, our calf, now a full-grown steer, was sent by rail or truck to the stockyards and consigned to a marketing firm for sale.

4. Buyers for several local and out-of-town meat packing companies put in bids based on the going consumer price of beef. This steer was one of a carload bought by an Ohio meat packing company.

5. At the packing plant, the "beef crew" turned beef on the hoof into meat for the store. Beef was inspected, chilled and graded, prepared for shipment.

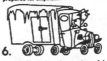

6. Under refrigeration, the quarters of beef were shipped to New York's wholesale meat district — 1500 miles from Texas, where the calf was born.

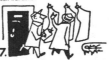

7. Owner of a Brooklyn meat market, after comparing prices and quality, selected a quarter of our steer.

8. In the store, a quarter of beef was turned into steaks, roasts, stew and hamburger; was displayed for customer's selection competing with other meats.

9. Yesterday, a housewife looked over everything in the counter, compared values, decided on steak, porterhouse or chopped, depending on what she wanted to spend.

**From *The Story of Beef*
The American Meat
Institute (Chicago).**

2

98

Upton Sinclair, in the book *The Jungle,* describes what really happens in meat packing plants. Meat eaters need to appreciate that animals are being injected with so many hormones that it is accelerating their growth. A chicken should take 16 weeks to reach full maturation; instead they are rushed into five weeks. The same applies to hogs and cattle.[3] They are herded into areas where they have no space to move. Cattle, chickens, hogs are literally placed in pens where there is no movement. The stench is unbelievable. They are placed on a conveyor belt to be slaughtered and the remaining parts off the conveyor belt are processed for bologna, salami, and hot dogs, and whatever else the meat packing plant can produce. Nothing is left to waste until it arrives in your body. A charcoal steak has as much benzopyrene, a carcinogen, as 600 cigarettes. If you must eat meat, consider organic and avoid barbecuing. This process produces carcinogenes. If you must use your grill invest in chemicals that can reduce some of its negative effects.

In the spirit of Thanksgiving, when the native Americans were saving the White man, Chief Seattle observed the treatment between the White man and animals. When the White man conquered the Native Americans, Chief Seattle had this humble request.

He did not ask something for himself, nor for his tribe, nor even for the Indian people. There were, of course, many things of immense importance he must have wanted at such a time. He could have asked for more blankets, horses, or food. He could have asked that the ancestral burial grounds be respected. He could have asked many things for himself or for his people. But what stood above all else in importance had to do with the relationship between humans and other animals. His one request was as prophetic as it was plain:

"I will make one condition,
The white man must treat the beasts of this land
As his brothers.
For whatever happens to the beasts
soon happens to man.
All things are connected."

Chief Seattle spoke for a people whose bond with the natural world was unimaginably profound. Yet the white man called them savages, and utterly disregarded his plea. The factory farms that produce today's meats, dairy products and eggs are living testimony to how totally we have disdained the one condition he made.

The White man thought Chief Seattle an ignorant savage. But he was a prophet whose wisdom and eloquence arose from living contact with Creation. And his words are astoundingly similar to those of a book written long, long ago. The *Bible,* too, tells us the fates of humans and animals are intimately intertwined.

"For that which befalleth the sons of men befalleth the beasts.
Even one thing befalleth them:
As the one dieth, so dieth the other;
Yea, they have all one breath,
So that a man hath no pre-eminence above a beast."[4]
(ECCLESIASTES 3:19)

As I continued to read about how animals are mistreated, I thought about how could a Christian who values life be so inhumane to animals? Because we live in an urban society, we are divorced from meat processing. Most of us don't make the connection between McDonalds and meat packing plants. For many of us, even if we theoretically knew, we are ruled by taste and not morality.

In an earlier chapter, we spoke about the amount of acreage and water required to produce a pound of meat in comparison to a pound of vegetables. There is no reason for any of the six billion people in the world to be hungry, unless we disproportionately allocate an excessive amount of land for the production of livestock.

One of the things that I just couldn't shake was when I read the different size of the intestine and colon for animals and humans. Animals are designed to kill meat, consume it, and evacuate it. We let someone else kill our meat, they inject chemicals, and we consume it six months later.

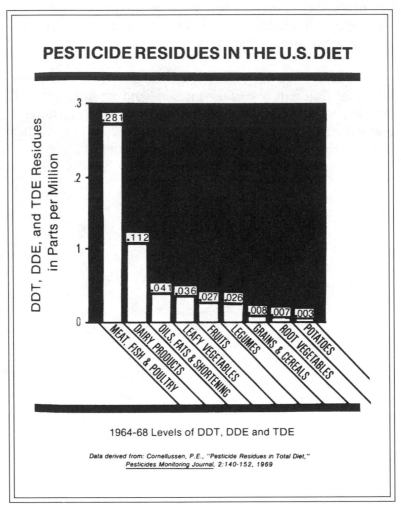

PESTICIDE RESIDUES IN THE U.S. DIET

DDT, DDE, and TDE Residues in Parts per Million

.281
.112
.041
.036
.027
.026
.008
.007
.003

MEAT, FISH & POULTRY
DAIRY PRODUCTS
OILS, FATS & SHORTENING
LEAFY VEGETABLES
FRUITS
LEGUMES
GRAINS & CEREALS
ROOT VEGETABLES
POTATOES

1964-68 Levels of DDT, DDE and TDE

Data derived from: Cornellussen, P.E., "Pesticide Residues in Total Diet," Pesticides Monitoring Journal, 2:140-152, 1969

5

If you look at the human intestine and the colon it is very long and intricate. We were designed to digest nutrients before evacuation. Meat stays for long periods of time. It is estimated pork stays in the small and large intestine and the colon approximately 12 to 14 days. What is unfortunate is that even with that estimate it does not mean all of the pork has been eliminated. The trichina worm cannot be eliminated. Unfortunately, the worms hatch within our intestines. This is one of the major reasons for stomach problems, headaches, and fatigue. Beef stays approximately 8 to 12 days, chicken 6 to 8 days, and fish 3 to 5 days. While many consider fish a good alternative to red meat, and it is a good source of Omega 3 oil, there are some consequences. There are 700 chemicals found in most seas including mercury. Fish are considered spoiled when the bacteria counts exceed 10 million per gram. Catfish has 27 million per gram. Fried fish destroys almost all nutrients.[6]

In contrast, fruits and vegetables can be digested and eliminated within six hours. In retrospect, if you look at the amount of time that a meat-eating animal takes to eliminate, it parallels the amount of time humans require to digest and eliminate fruits and vegetables. I don't think this is an accident. Our God is too awesome to operate on happenstance.

I continued to read and found that a vegetarian diet can prevent 97 percent of coronary problems.[7] It is highly unusual for a vegetarian to have high blood pressure, suffer a stroke, heart disease, arthritis, rheumatism, and cancer. That was enough for me. That night I made the second most important decision in my life and became a vegetarian. Obviously, the first was confessing Jesus as Lord of my life.

I would not recommend my approach to becoming a vegetarian. For most people, a better approach would be a gradual reduction of meat, from pork to beef to chicken to fish to vegetarianism. This is very similar to the approach we should take with fasting. Health experts recommend before fasting there should be a cleansing process. You don't go from chitterlings to carrot juice. The body needs to adjust to various stages. The other challenge that I had was being a college student living in a dormitory. I was not in control of my diet. Consequently, I became a non-meat eater not a vegetarian. There is a tremendous difference between a vegetarian and a non-meat eater.

Only five percent of the American population are vegetarians.[8] The two traditional classifications are vegetarians and lacto-ovo vegetarians who add dairy and eggs to their diet. But many vegetarians, including myself, for a period of time are non meat eaters. It is very easy for a non-meat eater to be unhealthy. It is very possible that a meat eater who understands basic nutritional principles could have a better diet than a non-meat eater. A non-meat eater could go to McDonald's and ask them to take the meat off the hamburger, but keep the white hamburger bun, processed cheese, iceberg lettuce, tomato with french fries, and a milk shake. Have you noticed that McDonald's french fries like so many others cannot be reheated? The food has been dead for a long time. This person is erroneously calling himself a vegetarian, but this meal has only two vegetables, a sliver of lettuce and a slice of tomato. I pointed out that iceberg lettuce is the lightest green lettuce in the lettuce family, which means it has very little chlorophyll. That type of diet does not bode well on your overall health. In comparison, a meat eater could have a lean piece of meat and a full salad and actually consume more nutrients than the non-meat eater.

What I have learned over the years is that to be a vegetarian requires not only a great degree of effort, perseverance and organizational skills, but a scientific knowledge of what the body requires daily. I am very much aware that as a vegetarian in a meat and sugar culture, I need to carry fruit, nuts, raisins, and granola bars. There is a very good chance at the airport, vending machine, and along the highways there may be no fruit or vegetables. A vegetarian diet is less expensive, requires little cleaning due to less fat, and almost total elimination of medicine and hospital bills.

One of the most important substances that our bodies need are enzymes. When I first became a vegetarian, I was not aware of the distinction between cooked and raw food. I did not make a distinction between boiling broccoli out of a can and eating raw broccoli. There is a tremendous difference between cooked food and raw food. Ideally speaking, 80 percent of our diet should be raw. When food is cooked almost 80 percent of the enzymes needed for digestion are lost. The American diet lends itself toward cooked food. It takes an even more conscious effort to have the bulk of your diet raw.

There are many non-meat eaters who consume a large amount of refined carbohydrates. As we mentioned in an earlier chapter, a non-meat eater who consumes a lot of cookies, cakes, pies and other refined carbohydrates filled with sugar could become a Type II diabetic. The consequences of being a diabetic resemble some of the same diseases of meat consumption. Can you imagine a vegetarian (non-meat eater) with high blood pressure dying of heart disease? A non-meat eater is a junk food eater. This explains why some vegetarians become overweight because of their large consumption of refined carbohydrates.

I have learned over the years that because the soil does not have the 103 minerals and vitamins that our bodies so desperately need, that it requires vitamin supplements. There was a period of time when I thought as a vegetarian if I consumed vegetables and fruit, that all of my vitamins and minerals would be secured. That line of thought would have been correct in the early 1900s. Whether we like it or not we must take vitamins.

Because our bodies are 80 percent water, we must consume more water. It is very possible for a meat eater to consume more water than a non meat eater. Vegetarians should know better. They should not only drink more, but know the water should be filtered, distilled, or boiled. I recommend distilled water because almost all minerals are removed. Critics of distilled water because it lacks minerals need to acknowledge that 95 percent of minerals consumed will come from food not water. The risk of consuming toxic inorganic chemicals is not worth the benefit of consuming tap or bottled water.

An incorrect assumption is that vegetarians are weaker, lack energy, stamina, and speed. I wonder if the vegetarian diet is affecting the speed of horses? I wonder if the vegetarian diet is affecting the strength of elephants? There have been numerous studies comparing vegetarians to meat eaters.

Professor Irving Fisher designed a series of tests to compare the stamina and strength of meat eaters to vegetarians. He selected men from three groups: meat eating athletes, vegetarian athletes, and vegetarian sedentary subjects. Fisher reported the results of his study in the Yale Medical Journal. His findings do not seem to lend a great deal of creditability that meat builds strength. Of the three groups compared, meat eaters showed far less endurance than the vegetarians, even when they were leading a sedentary life.

Overall, the average score of the vegetarians was over double the average score of the meat eaters, even though half of the vegetarians were sedentary people, while all of the meat eaters tested were athletes. After analyzing all of the factors that might have been involved in the results, Fisher concluded the difference in the endurance between flesh eaters and vegetarians was due entirely to diet.[9]

A comparable study was done by Dr. Jay Iotyko in Paris. He compared the endurance of vegetarians and meat eaters from all walks of life in a variety of tests. The vegetarians averaged two to three times more stamina than the meat eaters. Even more remarkably they took only 20 percent of the time to recover from exhaustion compared to their meat eating rivals.[10]

A Danish team of researchers tested a group of men on a variety of diets using a stationary bicycle to measure strength and endurance. The men were fed a mixed diet of meat and vegetables for a period of time and then tested on the bicycle. The average time they could peddle before muscle failure was 114 minutes. These same men at a later date were fed a high diet in meat, milk, and eggs for a similar period and then retested on the bicycles. On the high meat diet their peddling time before muscle failure dropped dramatically to an average of only 57 minutes. Later these same men were switched to a strictly vegetarian diet composed of grains, beans, vegetables and fruit and then tested on the bicycles. They peddled an average of 167 minutes. Wherever and whenever tests of this nature have been done, the results have been similar. Doctors in Belgium systematically compared the number of times vegetarians and meat eaters could squeeze a grip meter. The vegetarians won handily with an average of 69 while the meat eaters averaged only 38.[11]

I know of many other studies in the medical literature, which report similar findings, but I know of not one that has arrived at different results. The Seventh Day Adventists, who espouse vegetarianism, have a 72 percent less chance of incurring cancer.[12] A vegetarian diet reduces the length and severity of menstrual cramps. This is a result of less fat consumption which increases estrogen production.

As I continued to read various books on vegetarianism, I became more and more concerned about the relationship between meat intake, heart disease, and cancer. These are America's twin killers. The death rates have increased over the years while more and more money has been allocated for research. America seems to be adamant about reducing heart disease and cancer without reducing or eliminating meat.

One of the toughest questions I've ever been asked as a public speaker is how do you change someone's diet when diet is habitual? I believe the best way is to lead by example and provide alternatives.

Listed below is an alternative lifestyle chart.

Life threatening Foods	Life sustaining foods
White bread	Whole wheat or rye bread
Ice cream	Soy ice cream
Cow's milk	Human milk, sesame milk, soy milk
Cheese	Soy and tofu cheese
Meat	Soy bean products, beans, and tofu
Tap water	Distilled, spring, filtered, boiled water

Table salt	Himalayan Crystal Salt, Spike, Sea Salt
Chocolate	Carob
White Rice	Brown rice
White flour	Wheat or rye flour
Sugar	Molasses, unrefined honey
Junk food	Dried fruit, rice cakes, nuts, raisins, whole wheat pretzels, and unsalted potato chips
White macaroni and spaghetti	Whole-wheat macaroni and spaghetti
Pancakes	Buck wheat or whole wheat pancakes
Eggs	Egg substitutes

Many people ask me, "What do you eat? It seems such a restricted diet. There doesn't seem to be much variety." My first response is "there are more fruits and vegetables than meats." I then remember. I'm talking to someone who when asked what they are having for dinner only answers meat. For someone who has a meat obsession, a meal without meat is no meal at all.

I try to answer the question starting with breakfast. I may start with a glass of juice. I may eat individual pieces of fruit or make a fruit salad. I love starting the day with either a piece of watermelon, cantaloupe, honeydew melon, pineapples, or mango. Remember, the word breakfast is break the fast, and we should not break a fast with a ten pound meal that puts us to sleep. I also like making protein drinks combining juices, banana, spirulina, ginseng, and bee pollen. It gives me a energy boost. This is a great alternative for people who cannot function without caffeine. For those who are looking for something heavier we could have oatmeal, cream of wheat, or cereal as long as it's 100 percent grain with soy or sesame seed milk. We could also have buckwheat pancakes or waffles. If we wanted something a little heavier we could cook soy bean bacon or sausage, egg substitutes, potatoes, and whole wheat toast. For lunch we could have either a fruit or vegetable salad, soup, or a soybean sandwich. When our boys were younger, they would invite their friends over to the house and wouldn't tell them that they were eating soy bean hot dogs or hamburgers. Many of their friends had no idea what they were eating, but they knew it tasted good. For dinner, I may have a vegetable salad, baked potato, steamed vegetables, cabbage, greens, or beans. My favorite would be beans. Unfortunately, for many of us as our income as risen, bean consumption has decreased. When you eat beans and greens don't throw away the "pot liquor" which has many nutrients.

For snacks throughout the day, I could have nuts and raisins, granola, dried fruit, and granola bars. For dessert, I could have tofu or soy ice cream. We could make cookies from whole-wheat flour. I could also have additional fruit for dessert.

As we conclude this chapter, I want to remind you of the scripture "I placed before you blessings and curses, life and death, choose life." Do not make your lifestyle decision based on taste, habit, or peer pressure. Ask the Lord to guide you. "Trust in the Lord with all thy heart and lean not to thy own understanding, In all thy ways, acknowledge Him, and He will direct your path." The Lord will give you a spirit of discernment.

You will need this spirit as you enter the doctor's office and read the next chapter.

THE DOCTOR SAID!

The "son" of medicine, Hippocrates acknowledges the "father" and founder is Imhotep. In the Hippocratic oath he acknowledges Imhotep using his Greek name Aesculapius. Imhotep was born approximately 2800 BC while Hippocrates was born near 500 BC. Hippocrates studied in Egypt.[1]

Imhotep believed the physician should "cause no harm". A doctor before prescribing drugs and considering surgery should remember the teachings of Imhotep. He also taught that food should be your medicine and medicine be your food.

The Chinese, who also have a very ancient tradition, believe that the superior physician teaches people to sustain their health. In rural China, doctors are paid when you are well.[2] That's a tremendous shift in paradigm. In most countries, including America, doctors are paid when you are sick. If doctors empowered patients and taught them preventive care they would not be paid. In China, health care is less expensive to deliver and they prefer to call it self care verses sick care. They prefer to call their clinics wellness centers. In China herbs, acupuncture, and energy balance are all extremely important. The concept of energy "Qi gong" is based on the belief that if your energy is strong no illness can befall you.

I believe American doctors are the best in the world if you have a gun shot wound or automobile accident. I believe that we have the best emergency room facilities in the world. The problem is that your chances of dying from a gun shot wound or an automobile accident are minute compared to your chances of dying from what you ate at the kitchen

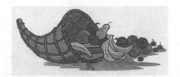
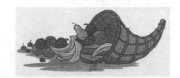

111

table. That creates the dilemma. If the two leading reasons for death—heart disease and cancer—are a result of lifestyle, then we need a medical profession who understands and appreciates the significance of nutrition.

The problem is only 30 of the 125 medical schools in the United States have a single required course in nutrition. A senate investigation revealed that the average physician in the United States received less than three hours of training in nutrition during four years of medical school.[3] This is one of the most significant statements in this book. Our health is in the hands of professionals who have less than three hours of training in nutrition! I won't even phantom what they were taught in those three hours. The nutrition class could have been sponsored by the pork, beef, chicken, fish, and dairy associations. This explains why many doctors do not appreciate fasting, colonics, enemas, vitamins, herbs, exercise, vegetarianism, acupuncture, and other alternative treatment.

I have reserved the following chapter on natural healing to look at these factors. This chapter is reserved for the medical profession and their healing methods. Let me jokingly say as you've heard often in Black and White relationships, "Some of my best friends are doctors." I love and respect them dearly and they have a tremendous amount of intelligence. Many of them were my classmates. They had a burning desire to make a difference. Many of them are very frustrated about an industry that is now controlled by the insurance companies, the courts, and the pharmaceutical industry.

Many of them had to leave the medical profession because they could not pay the insurance premiums. Many doctors who have brilliant minds resent that they have become pill distributors. As the country moves more into HMO's, many African American doctors are being squeezed out of their practices. More will be said about that in a subsequent chapter on racism.

I mentioned earlier it is better to see a sermon than to hear one. As a patient, I would be concerned if my doctor was overweight, out of shape, and suffering either from high blood pressure, diabetes, arthritis, rheumatism, heart disease, or cancer. Unfortunately, doctors have one of the lowest levels of life expectancy of any careers.

The health care industry is a trillion dollar industry.[4] Pharmaceutical companies spend 1.5 billion dollars on advertising. It represents 17 percent of the US economy. Each American spends $3,925.00 a year on health care.[5] More than 44 million Americans lack health insurance, leaving the country with the dubious distinction of having the most technologically advanced—but least equitable—health care system in the industrialized world.[6] Many people who have entertained the idea of quitting their jobs and becoming entrepreneurs have had second thoughts because they were unable to pay for health care. The pharmaceutical industry annually releases 13,000 new drugs.

Receiving the wrong medication, a bad reaction to the medication, or the wrong combination is now the sixth leading cause of death in America. Depending upon whose research you accept, between 100,000 on the low side and 300,000 on the high side die because of a misdiagnosis on medicine. Twenty-eight percent of patients hospitalized are there because of the above.[7]

The famous doctor Sir William Ossler said, "The desire to take medicine is perhaps the greatest failure which distinguishes man from animals." If you notice in the animal kingdom when an animal is not feeling well they go off by themselves and fast. When they feel a little better they eat grass. They know the power of chlorophyll. They don't have to be taught; it's their nature. God has given man dominion over the earth. We have the highest level of intelligence and yet when we get ill we go to a medical profession that has less than three hours of training in nutrition who over prescribes drugs, and we spend almost $4,000 a year. Are animals smarter than humans?

Thirteen percent of the population, primarily those over 65, consume one-third of all drugs. Can doctors cure without drugs? Do drugs really cure? Do drugs address the root problem? In America there seems to be contradictions; capitalism is king. Drugs stores will sell pharmaceutical drugs in one aisle and liquor and cigarettes in another.

I mentioned previously that HMO's and the pharmaceutical industry are controlling many doctors. Many of the pharmaceutical companies provide incentives to doctors, i.e. extra vacations, cruises, and other financial incentives if they prescribe their drugs. *60 Minutes* aired on December 19, 1999 the tremendous pressure pharmaceutical companies are placing on doctors and research universities. Many doctors are threatened if they question the success of a drug or its higher price over an equally qualified generic drug. Forty-one million drugs are prescribed weekly by OBGYN's and internists. Pediatricians and family doctors prescribe a greater number than the above just for ear infections.[8] Antibiotics kill bacteria not the virus.

Let me describe the drug treadmill in America. A healthy 50-year-old man visits his doctor for an annual checkup and is prescribed a seemingly harmless drug Tagamet for indigestion. Tagamet causes his joints pain, but he does not know it is the Tagamet. He starts to take Tylenol to treat the pain. He likes to have a few cocktails before dinner and he doesn't know that combining alcohol and Tylenol can cause serious damage (liver damage caused by Tylenol is one of the leading causes of emergency visits in the United States). In addition the Tagamet is already putting stress on the liver. His liver is being chronically damaged. Because of the constant stress his liver is unable to keep up with detoxifying the body, and soon he is coming down with colds and getting infections. The doctor prescribes antibiotics which further compromise the immune system and cause damage to the intestines. Furthermore, he now has a chronic sinus infection for which he takes allergy drugs that makes him irritable. This is a typical scenario of what is happening to many American patients. Remember Imhotep's motto, "Cause no harm."

Here's a typical scenario of how this unholy drug HMO alliance is playing itself across America. Let's take a typical 63-year-old woman named Ann who goes to her HMO for an annual check up carrying her bag of pills. She is already on the drug treadmill taking an ACE inhibitor to lower her blood pressure, which is marginally high. A cough suppressant to treat the nagging cough that is caused by the ACE inhibitor, sleeping pills to help her sleep because her cough keeps waking her. The estrogen Premarin for hormone replacement therapy, the synthetic progesterone primavera to offset the cancer promoting effect of the estrogen, which along with the sleeping pills makes her tired and mentally foggy. The anti-osteoporosis drug Fosamax which is giving her heartburn, Tagamet to treat the heart burn, and Metamucil to treat the constipation and indigestion caused because the Tagamet is suppressing her stomach acid, which was low. Ann isn't feeling too great, but she has been reading more about natural health and has decided that she wants to come off her drugs, replacing them with a lifestyle change. She's hoping her physician will help her with a weight loss program to lower her blood pressure and a natural progesterone cream for her osteoporosis and hormone replacement therapy. She also plans to use psyllium instead of Metamucil until her constipation goes away, and plans to use Melotonin if her increased exercise doesn't help with sleep. She has a list of what she wants to do and eagerly brings it to her physician.

The typical medical visit has you sitting in the waiting room for your scheduled appointment. You are brought in 30 minutes after you were scheduled. You are placed in a small observation room and told to undress and place this gown over you. You then wait another 10 or 15 minutes because this is also taking place with 3 other patients simultaneously. The doctor who is known as God by many patients arrives. You want to tell your doctor about the above scenario and your desire to reduce the medication. The doctor tells you she doesn't know about the "hocus pocus" natural stuff and if you want to continue being treated by your HMO you need to cooperate and take the drugs prescribed. You plead that since you started on these drugs life is hardly worth living. You're tired, coughing, and depressed.

The doctor brushes you off saying, "Everything in the bag is approved by the HMO." If you have any health complications caused by doing something different than prescribed your insurance might not cover it or your rate will increase. This scares you. What if you need surgery and your physician claims it was caused because you did not follow instructions. "Ok," you say, "I'll take the drugs. But I looked up the ACE inhibitor I'm taking and it says one of its common side effects is a nagging cough. Couldn't you put me on a different drug to lower my blood pressure?" Her physician impatiently pulls out a chart and quickly scans it and says, This is the drug approved by this HMO for your problem, I'm afraid you will have to live with it." This happens too many times in America.

Two hundred and seventy five million doctor visits are due to high blood pressure. One of eleven Americans suffers from high blood pressure. Three of the most pre-scribed drugs are acetaminophen, better known as Tylenol, ibuprofen, and aspirin.[9]

DRUG	ACTION	SIDE AFFECTS
Tylenol	Relieves pain, reduces fever	Liver and kidney damage, rash and dizziness
Aspirin	Reduces fever, relieves pain, reduces inflammation	Allergic reaction, stomach upset gastrointestinal bleeding, ulcers, ringing ears, should not be used by pregnant women or children
Ibuprofen (Advil)	Reduces fever, relieves pain, effective for menstrual pain, reduces inflammation	Skin rashes, itching, stomach upset and digestive problems

Aspirin is so popular it does not require prescription. Thirty million Americans have chronic headaches, and twenty million have occasional headaches. The biggest cause of headaches is a bad reaction to drugs followed by constipation, thyroid problems, high blood pressure, hypoglycemia, and caffeine withdrawal.[10] I have been fortunate that since I became a vegetarian I have not had a headache in three decades.

One of the more popular prescriptions for high blood pressure is diuretic. This creates a greater desire to urinate. The problem is that while it's working on decreasing the blood pressure, it also creates a greater desire to urinate. The problem with greater urination is that you are also losing valuable minerals, which are needed by the body.

Another major area where drugs are prescribed is in the area of flu. Every fall Americans are put through the annual flu season vaccination ritual. The ritual goes like this, you go to your physician and he/she tells you the flu can be deadly, and that a flu shot will prevent it. You get the shot and feel terrible for a week, and then a couple of months later you get the flu along with everyone else. The next year rolls around and you ask yourself should I or shouldn't I get a flu shot? Deaths from flu are increasing in spite of flu shots. According to statistics by the Center for Disease Control the death rate increased 59 percent since 1979. Even adjusting for a population increase there is still a 44 percent increase in deaths related to pneumonia and influenza.[11]

If flu vaccinations are working so well why is this happening? One reason is that as you age, which is when you need the most protection from flu, your body's ability to create anti-bodies to the vaccine deteriorates. Because the

118

flu virus is different every year, the flu shot will only be pro-
tective if the manufacturers of the vaccine are lucky enough
to pick the right flu virus!

A study from the Netherlands shows that among two
groups of elderly people, one that received flu shots and one
that received a placebo, the group receiving the flu shot only
had a one percent lower incidence of flu then the placebo
group![12]

I am equally concerned about the million plus children who are receiving Ritalin because they are diagnosed as
being hyperactive. You would think that in this sugar conscious society where children are consuming over 155 pounds
of sugar and before prescribing Ritalin doctors would recommend reducing if not eliminating sugar from the diet. Unfortunately, doctors and the pharmaceutical industry do not
make money with a change in diet and sugar reduction. The
four major reasons for children's visits are attention deficit
disorder (ADD), earaches, asthma, and obesity.[13] Should children receive drugs or a change in diet?

Ironically one third of all drugs come from plants,
yet the pharmaceutical industry is resistant to herbs. I have
not read research where someone died using nutritional
supplements. My major concern is how can a person be poi-
soned back to health? I also don't believe that doctors spend
four years in college and four years of medical school and
two years of residency to be drug dealers. Doctors need to
look in the mirror and honestly ask themselves am I doing
what is best for my patient or am I now an agent for the
HMO and pharmaceutical industry?

My concern is that too many doctors have acquiesced and
have felt that the HMO's and the pharmaceutical industries

are Goliaths. Doctors need to read the *Bible* and find out David defeated Goliath! One doctor who made that decision was Dr. James Balch. He said, "I knew that most of the men I was operating on with prostate problem would probably never have sex again. Finally I just couldn't do it anymore, I knew there must be a better way."

We are moving to a point where it will be hard to find anyone over 70 without prostate disease. American doctors perform 150,000 radical prostatectomies annually. In contrast, Sweden does 150 annually. The major side effect of surgery is impotence in 85 percent and 65 percent of men will be incontinent, dripping urine and wearing pads for the rest of their lives.[14] In a July 1997 study, noted in the Journal of Urology, men who had radiation implant treatment for localized prostate cancer had a failure rate of 86 percent with recurrence of cancer within 5 years.[15]

Because the medical profession is an equal opportunity destroyer, women should not feel exempt. There are 750,000 hysterectomies performed annually. Some researchers estimate that 650,000 are unnecessary.[16] The second best choice to vegetarian diet would be a hysteroscopy or myomectomy where only the fibroids are removed and the uterus is maintained. I also recommend a lumpectomy versus a radical mastectomy. The former surgeries are more time consuming and many doctors consider their extra effort over your organs. In a subsequent chapter on *The Health Legacy of Slavery and Racism* we will look at fibroids. African Americans disproportionately experience hysterectomies as doctors rationalize this as the most effective approach to removing fibroids.

In Europe, doctors are not as drug and surgery ori-
ented as American doctors. Europeans are more open to natural medicines, which may be the reason for greater life expectancy. Europe's success in curing and relieving prostate
problems has been much higher than America. For example,
most German doctors won't even consider the American approach. Similar attitudes exist in France and other European
countries.[17]

With heavy pharmaceutical advertising, vitamins and
herbs have very little chance of capturing the imagination of
most Americans. I would be careful in a capitalistic country
were money is king and many doctors have succumbed to
selecting surgery over other options, because it is financially
lucrative. It's not a tough financial decision for many doctors choosing between vitamins, herbs, diet, and exercise
versus a $50,000 surgery.

I pray that we never have another doctor who makes
the decision based on money or ignorance. With cancer killing one of three Americans, we have to ask ourselves is there
really a war on cancer? How can we spend billions of dollars
on research and the figure rise? Why was it only 1 of 33
dying of cancer in the early 1900s without research? Do
surgery, chemotherapy, and radiation remove the reason for
cancer occurring? The issue is not the tumor; the tumor is a
metabolic imbalance. What created the imbalance that produced the tumor? Surgery, chemotherapy, and radiation do
not address those questions. Our medical profession reminds
me of cowboys and Indians. We believe we can cure cancer
with a radiation gun, surgical knife, and chemotherapy. The
American medical profession uses a left-brain linear approach
to solve health problems. They believe if you have an ailment, they can offer a specific drug to address the problem.

God's body cannot be isolated like that. Our bodies should be viewed from a "holistic" approach. The ailment is a reflection of an overall problem. The treatment must address toxicity and nutritional imbalance. There are many diseases, but all cures begin with detoxification.

In the following chapter on natural healing, we will look at alternatives to the medical profession for both heart disease and cancer. If you think I am critical of the medical profession, I am more concerned about patients blindly accepting everything they say! My concern is that God gave our bodies to us not doctors, yet many of us across demographics have relinquished full responsibility of our health to a professional who has three hours of nutritional training. I have lost too many friends and relatives who gave complete control of their health care to doctors. My wife and I have given tons of information to family members and friends for them to make an informed decision.

As a CEO of my company, I hire lawyers and accountants and other professionals to perform a particular function. How can I hire them if I do not know the issues? I need to know enough about the area to ask appropriate questions. I also need to know when I hear the correct answer.

The same thing applies in the medical profession. How can a patient have dialogue with a doctor, who only gives them 15 minutes with limited nutritional background and pressured by HMO's and pharmaceutical companies? Secondly, how can you participate in a discussion if you know very little about the function of your liver, kidney, heart, and the rest of your organs? What will be the quality of the conversation if you don't know the significance of the 103 vitamins and nutrients your body requires?

One of the major catalysts for writing this book is that I got tired of friends and relatives telling me what the doctor said. My reaction was what did you say? It's your health, what do you say? Can you imagine my friends and relatives asking a doctor can they take carrot juice, can they take wheatgrass, can they fast or have an enema or colonic? Can you imagine someone asking a doctor about reducing his or her meat consumption if not eliminating it or considering eating more raw food? What is worse is when the doctors say no to wheatgrass and carrot juice and the patient accepts it! The patient has absolute trust in the doctor, no questions asked. They really believe the doctor is going to save them. The answer is in the pill, knife, and radiation. Unfortunately, many Americans have never made a health decision; it was always done by the doctor. Research indicates that patients who use alternative treatments do not inform their doctors because they feel their doctor is unwilling, disinterested, and will give a negative response.[18]

Unfortunately, after they have done everything the doctor wanted them to do, the doctor announces to the patient and family that we have done everything we can do, and you have less than three months to live. Many patients still do not second guess themselves and do not pursue alternative treatment. Satan has convinced them it would be better to die than to be disappointed with alternative treatment. Others try, but unfortunately it was too late. Surgery had removed organs, and radiation and chemotherapy had destroyed the immune system; therefore it was too late.

For my mother, they performed surgery and removed the gallbladder. The doctors never discussed with the family what created hundreds of gallstones. It is very difficult digesting without a gall bladder. I now know that gall stones can be removed without surgery. If you drink one quart of apple juice daily for five days, this will soften the stones. On the sixth day fast, take a tablespoon of Epson Salt with water, follow four hours later with four ounces of olive oil and fresh lemon juice. In the morning you will eliminate the gall stones.[19] Again, does chemotherapy and radiation address why the tumor existed? They found tumors and used the combination of chemotherapy and radiation. This destroyed her immune system.

The state is willing to pay for patients to be transported to clinics and hospitals to receive drugs and surgery, but if a family prefers alternative treatment, there is little to no funding or transportation to visit chiropractors and naturopaths, and receive herbs, vitamins, and colonics.

Never let a doctor rush you into making a decision about surgery, radiation, or chemotherapy. The decision could be irreversible and unnecessary. I strongly suggest you consult a natural healer for a second opinion before making a final decision. I could give you horror stories of doctors who have taken families to court who did not agree with their recommended treatment. They wanted the spouse, parent, relative, or guardian to be considered unfit. Can you imagine, here you are fighting for the health of a loved one and now you have to fight the courts? I pray for the day that doctors will be genuinely interested in patients who were cured naturally. Many doctors do not learn from their patients who were healed with alternative treatments. I have seen doctors deny that cancer existed if the patient used other means for healing.

I look forward to the day when doctors and hospitals will offer carrot juice, vitamins, herbs, and workout facilities.

We should visit doctors not just when we are sick, but when we are well. They should encourage prevention not drugs. I would love for my doctor to recommend buying a treadmill. I would enjoy a doctor giving me vitamin C, recommending fasting, enemas, colonics. I would like to see the emphasis on prevention. My greatest desire is for patients to be empowered. My prayer is that you never enter another doctor's office until you thoroughly understand your body and your medical concerns. You should only select a doctor if he or she is willing to have a dialogue with you about your concerns, with the emphasis on drug-free prevention. I would also like for you to ask your doctor what are their views on nutrition? How many courses have you taken in nutrition?

In closing, I'm even more concerned about patients who not only accept what the doctor says on the front end of the treatment, but after the doctor has pronounced you dead while you are still living, we still not have asked what does God say? I believe that God has the final say. He is the best doctor and you need to ask your doctor, do you have a personal relationship with Jesus Christ? Can you imagine going under the knife of a surgeon who is not anointed with the Holy Spirit?

While this chapter has focused on doctors, I would strongly suggest that you no longer allow your dentist to fill cavities and root canals with mercury, which is extremely toxic and causes cancer and heart disease. Germany has banned mercury fillings. I encourage you to replace mercury fillings and all subsequent fillings with ceramic. If your dentist will not change, please contact a holistic dentist at the Environmental Dental Association at 1-800-388-8124.

In the following chapter on Divine Natural Healing we will look at alternative strategies to the medical profession. It is an answer to my prayer.

DIVINE NATURAL HEALING
(Healing begins with faith.)

This in my opinion is the most important chapter of the book. It will determine life or death. It will determine our faith. I pray that the following event never happens in your life. You walk into the doctor's office; you've been experiencing some degree of pain and discomfort. You have delayed this meeting for several weeks, but you know it's time to visit the doctor. You walk into his/her office and after a battery of tests the doctor informs you that you have a life threatening disease. They recommend surgery and an extensive amount of drugs. You return home.

The previous chapter was *"The Doctor Said!"* and the doctor has now spoken. My first question to you, what would God say? This is a terrible time for many people who did not have a relationship with Jesus. This is not the time not to have full command of the *Bible.* This is not the time to lack understanding of your body, the nature of the disease, and alternative treatment. Unfortunately, for many of us when we are in the doctor's office it is not a conversation, but a monologue. That is a result of a patient who does not know his or her rights or responsibilities.

My first recommendation in the above scenario is the decision should be delayed. You need to hear from the Lord, study your body, understand the disease, and look for alternative treatment. The Lord does not give us a spirit of fear. Fear should not dictate your decision. The Lord gives a spirit of power and love and sound mind. You will need all of the above to make a godly decision. You need to put Satan under your feet. You need to tell Satan he is a liar.

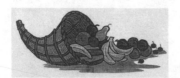 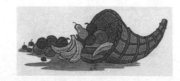

127

You should have full command of healing scriptures. I suggest making a healing tape. You need to create posters with these scriptures and mount them on your bedroom wall. Ideally these scriptures should have been internalized before you got to the "11th" hour, but God can heal at midnight.

You need to tell Satan I'm taking back my health. Tell him he can have his arthritis, rheumatism, heart disease, high blood pressure, strokes, diabetes, and cancer. Mark 11:23–24, reminds us to speak to the mountain. You need to believe in your heart that what you confess will happen. For the scripture reminds us whatever you believe in your heart will happen. In Hebrews 4:16, the Bible says, "Come boldly to the throne of grace, to obtain mercy and grace in the time of need." This is not the time to be a wimpish passive Christian. This is the time to call in your inheritance, that you are a joint heir with Jesus and heir to the throne. You have rights. God wants you to prosper in all things, including your health as your soul prospers.

How unfortunate that we have so many impotent Christians who have been "in church" for decades, but never "in Christ." They have been in the building, but not in His presence. They have worshipped in the sanctuary, but never made God Lord of their health, wealth, and sex life.

Psalm 103:3 says Who heals all your diseases. Don't call cancer the Big C. This is reserved for Christ. Christ is the big C. Cancer is the little c. Don't limit God. When the doctor says you have three months, what does God say? When the doctor gives you fatal news, read Luke 1:37, "With God nothing is impossible," when doctors say it is impossible for Him. Remember in Philippians 4:13, "I can do all things through Christ who strengthens me." I can overcome arthritis, rheumatism, heart disease, stroke, high blood pressure, diabetes, and cancer.

When you have the vision of your Savior on the Cross, and you are reminded of I Peter 2:24 "Who himself bore our sins in His own body on the tree, that we having died to sins might live for righteousness, by whose stripes you are healed. You need to claim your victory by His stripes. The victory had already been won. The scripture said "were" healed, therefore it is a mistake to say, "if" God heals me or He "will" heal me. All you have to do is claim your inheritance.

There are numerous faith stories in the Bible that illustrate people who were given the same prognosis, but knew God who said, "He would never leave them nor forsake them." I am reminded of Jacob in Genesis 32:6 who told God, "I will not let you go until you bless me."

I am reminded of the bleeding woman in Matthew 9:20–22, "And suddenly a woman who had a flow of blood for 12 years, came from behind and touched the hem of his garment. For she said to herself, If only I may touch His garment I shall be made well, but Jesus turned around and when He saw her He said, "Be of good cheer daughter, your faith has made you well," and the woman was made well from that hour. Do you have her faith? God needs faith only the size of a mustard seed.

I am reminded in Luke 18:38, 40–43, "Then he cried out saying, Jesus, son of David have mercy on me. So Jesus stood still and commanded him to be brought to Him. And when he came near, He asked him what do you want me to do for you? He said Lord that I may receive my sight and Jesus said to him receive your sight, your faith has made you well, and immediately he received his sight and followed him glorifying God." This blind man knew that if he could just talk to Jesus, he would be healed. He was bold, he spoke loud, he wasn't quiet. At this point in your life you don't need to be quiet or passive. You need to be bold and loud.

I'm reminded of the lepers in Luke 17:12–14. Then He entered a certain village and there met him 10 men who were lepers who stood far off and they lifted up their voices and said, "Jesus master have mercy on us." So when he saw them, He said to them "Ago, show yourself to the priest, and so it was as they went they were cleansed."

In that scripture, Jesus wanted to find out the level of their faith, so he told them to go show themselves to the priest. The Priest was not going to see them if they were not healed. The lepers knew that, but they believed Jesus. Jesus said go see the priest and that's what the lepers did. On their way to the priest Jesus healed them, but it was walking by faith that healed them.

I can't stress enough in this chapter, it is not what the doctors said, but what the Lord said. Do you believe God can heal you? Do you believe that He came to give you life, and to give you life more abundantly? Do you believe God is the best doctor? The last scripture that I want to share comes from Matthew 17:21. Jesus says, "However this kind does not go out except by prayer and fasting."

I love it when the medical community finally admits there is power in prayer. A study was done with 1,000 heart disease patients. Five hundred received prayer and the others did not. The group receiving prayer had significantly less complications.

There may come a time in your life when you have an illness that will only come out with prayer and fasting. The Bible reminds us that in II Corinthian 10:4 "For the weapons of our warfare are not carnal, but mighty in God for pulling down strongholds." You have an army that consists of the word, prayer, angels, fasting, and the Holy Spirit. Do you have a prayer partner? You must find another saint, touch and agree, for Jesus reminds us whatever you bind on earth, He will bind in Heaven. If two or three are gathered in my name, I shall be there also. For it is not by power, it is not by might, but it is by the Holy Spirit. These are your five weapons described in detail in Ephesians 6. You need to put on the full armor of God. Ideally speaking you had on the armor when entering the doctor's office. The role of the church in your healing is discussed in the last chapter.

The first phase of healing begins in the spiritual. The second phase is in the natural. Your weapons are chiropractors, naturopaths, herbalists, colon therapists, alternative treatment centers, juice therapy, vitamins, herbs, enemas, colonics, acupuncture, and much more. Wheatgrass is the best source in your healing process. You need to drink two to eight ounces throughout the day. Do not let any inconvenience deny you from healing. Cleaning the juicer or going to the juice bar is minuscule compared to death. Chiropractors believe in healing without drugs and surgery by working with the spinal cord. There are over 60,000 chiropractors in America and 20 million Americans are taking advantage of their service. There are 3,000 naturopaths who believe in fasting, nutrition, exercise, acupuncture, and herbal therapy. Colon therapists believe life and death are determined by the state of the colon. They provide colonics. Herbalists believe healing can be secured naturally with herbs not drugs.

I like to look at these types of healers as the first choice, not the alternative. I think we have it backwards. We give our lives to the medical profession first and after surgery and radiation and chemotherapy has been unsuccessful then we consider the above as an alternative. I would like for natural healing to be considered first and surgery, drugs, and radiation the alternative.

Let me put this into a scientific perspective. You have been diagnosed with cancer. You have a malignant tumor and surgery at best will only remove the tumor. Surgery, chemotherapy and radiation do not address the major question—why was the body unable to destroy cancerous cells? Many of us were unaware we have carried cancerous cells all of our lives. Our immune system has always been able to destroy those cells. Each one of us daily produces several hundred thousand cancer cells. Whether we develop clinical cancer or not depends upon the ability of our immune system to destroy cancer cells. Cancer thrives in a deficient immune system. Surgery, radiation, and chemotherapy at best destroy tumors. Unfortunately, they also destroy the immune system. You don't need a search and destroy mission. You need a healing therapy that will build your immune system.

Many people with heart disease are recommended by doctors to undergo bypass surgery. The cost of this procedure often exceeds $100,000 and possesses an eight percent risk factor. This surgery does not address the root problem—clogged arteries. Chelation therapy binds toxic metals and minerals from the body's tissues and eliminates them through the kidneys. This treatment is very inexpensive and 300 times safer. Could the reason that many doctors don't recommend chelation therapy be cost? Lack of knowledge?

The same thing is true with "catching a cold," which can only happen if you have a deficient immune system. Each and every day we are exposed to viruses and bacteria that can be detrimental to our bodies. The majority of the time our immune system is strong enough to fight them and we don't catch cold. But if our bodies are filled with mucus, which primarily comes from eating dead food or dairy products, then our immune system is unable to fight off the virus and the bacteria. We then make the mistake of giving ourselves anti-biotic, Nyquil, and other drugs because we want to suppress the cleansing process. What the body is trying to do is rid itself of waste. Ideally speaking, the waste would be eliminated through the colon or through the glands when exercising, sweating, using steam rooms, or saunas.

For many of us because of the foods consumed, we are tremendously constipated. The immune system is weakened during constipation. Many of us do not sweat, therefore the body knows no other way to rid itself of mucus than through the nasal passages commonly called a cold. We think by giving our bodies drugs that the problem is resolved. Most drugs in 72 hours or less stop the running nose. We think we stopped the cold, only to experience in the following weeks or months a more serious illustration of the body trying to cleanse, with a cough, bronchitis, or pneumonia.

You often see the signs during the construction season: we apologize for this short term inconvenience for a long term improvement. The same applies with cleansing the body. It is better to let the cold run its course and experience a short term inconvenience for a long term gain. This does not mean that you should not take anything, but you should not suppress the body's desire to rid itself of waste. Your cold was a result of excess mucous and the inability of your immune system to remove it through the colon or glands. During this cleansing, the solution is not drugs, but reducing mucous producing foods and building the immune system primarily with vitamins C, A, zinc, and echinacea.

The same is applicable with a fever. Your body is trying to burn waste that was unable to be eliminated through the colon. If you continue to feed your body dead food all that does is increase the fire. You would think that if you understood your body is on fire, you would reduce or eliminate food being burned, and would fast and consume more water.

Enemas, colonics, steam rooms, and saunas are excellent for colds and fevers.

The foundation of the natural healing approach is that illness is a result of toxic waste in the body. It can be seen in the blood stream and the colon. In an earlier chapter, we mentioned that your health is determined by the quality of your blood, and the state of your arteries and colon. When you visit chiropractors, naturopaths, and herbalists they help you develop a plan to detoxify your body. The three primary organs to be "flushed" are the kidneys, liver, and the colon.

The foundation of a detox program is fasting, juice therapy, vitamins, herbs, enemas, and colonics. Many Americans who are addicted to sugar, caffeine, alcohol, nicotine, and meat may experience withdrawal pains for a few days while detoxing. You are on the verge of healing! Do not let Satan take away your victory by convincing you it is better to return to your addictions. Satan will attack the weakest part of your body.

For many people fasting is just too demanding. They have never fasted before. They would choose surgery, radiation, and chemotherapy over fasting. Unfortunately for many of us we have never fasted. For many of us we have never missed a meal. And so in the 11th hour it becomes difficult for some of us to fast. That's why ideally speaking before you would enter that doctor's office for that dreadful news it would have been nice if you would have had some experience fasting. For many people they feel fasting is just too demanding, the requirements too great. I would choose fasting over surgery, radiation, and chemotherapy any day of the week. The Bible says, "Deny yourself, pick up your cross and follow Me." We must push ourselves, pick up your cross and follow Him. We must push ourselves away from the kitchen table. We could save $4,000 annually in drugs if we disciplined ourselves with fasting. Our lord and Savior fasted as much as 40 days. A good diet, juice therapy, vitamins, herbs, enemas, and colonics should be a necessity for the 44 million uninsured Americans and those who prefer "health care" over "sick care."

Detoxing requires fasting, juice therapy, vitamins, herbs, enemas, and colonics. Listed below are the various herbs and nutrients to address particular ailments. Find your particular problem and secure those nutrients and begin to feel better. Wheatgrass, carrot-beet-spinach juice, vitamins A, C, and E should be taken daily.

AILMENTS	HERBS AND VITAMINS
Acne/Skin	Chaparral, dandelion, echinacea
Adrenals	Licorice
AIDS	Golden seal, pau d'arco, echinacea, garlic, rose hips, combine with a colon cleanser (e.g. cascara sagrada, senna or psyllium)
Alertness (Staying Awake)	Ginseng, ginkgo, gota kola, licorice root, oil of lemon (inhale)
Alcoholic Habit (Abuse)	Licorice, dandelion
Allergies/Sinus	Bayberry, bee pollen; clean blood with yellowdock, burdock or other blood cleanser.
Arterioscleroses	Garlic, capsicum, hawthorn
Alzheimers	Gota kola, lecithin, ginkgo
Anemia	Kelp, spirulina, iron supplement: also prunes, sunflower seeds, figs
Appendix Problems	Buckthorn, cascara sagrada
Appetite (Improve)	Alfalfa, chamomile, peppermint, fennel
Appetite (Reduce)	Spirulina, chickweed, fennel

Arthritis	Alfalfa, burdock, comfrey, yucca; eat no animal products
Asthma	Mullein and Lobelia (taken together), chamomile, barberry, hyssop, comfrey: herba santa
Atherosclerosis	Garlic, cayenne; ecithin
Athlete's Foot	Chamomile, safflower; clean colon
Back Sprain	Comfrey and valerian (together)
Bed Wetting	Cornsilk, uva ursi, peach bark
Bladder Infection	Juniper berries, cornsilk, plantain
Blood Poisoning	Echinacea, chickweed, golden seal
Blood Pressure	Cayenne, garlic, hyssop
Blood Purifiers	Burdock (arthritis); dandelion (liver, addictions, and build the blood); chaparral (skin); echinacea (entire body), garlic, red clover
Boils	Echinacea, garlic, golden seal
Bones	Comfrey, horsetail; also eat foods and take supplements rich in vitamin C and the mineral calcium
Brain	Gota kola, blessed thistle, ginkgo
Bronchitis	Comfrey, eucalyptus, lobelia, cayenne
Bruises	Comfrey, cayenne, dandelion, lavender (apply topically)
Burns	Aloe vera; a good salve (topical for healing)
Bursitis	Alfalfa, chaparral, comfrey
Caffeine Addiction	Licorice, dandelion
Cancer/Tumor	Pau D'arco, golden seal, echinacea; chaparral and red clover combination; don't eat animal products, drink fruit (e.g. lemons) and vegetable (e.g. carrot) juices
Cancer Sore	Myrrh, golden seal
Cataracts	Chaparral, eyebright, gota kola

136

Chicken Pox	Golden seal, echinacea; also eat no animal products
Child Birth (Before)	raspberry, squawvine
Child Birth (After)	Red raspberry
Childhood Disease	Golden seal, echinacea; yarrow, rosehips and licorice (together)
Cholesterol	Echinacea, hawthorn berries
Circulation	Cayenne, garlic, golden seal
Cleanser (General Body)	Garlic, golden seal
Colds	Astragalus, peppermint, lemon grass, mullein, bayberry
Colds Hands or Feet	Cayenne, sage
Colitis	Comfrey, slippery elm
Colon	Senna, Cascara sagrada, aloe vera, or psyllium
Constipation	Burdock, red clover, (mild constipation); psyllium, cascara sagrada, senna, aloe vera (severe constipation)
Cracked Lips	Parsley, garlic, fenugreek
Dandruff	Anise, rosemary, Jojoba oil
Diabetes	Dandelion, golden seal, uva ursi; intelligent eating and exercise
Diarrhea	Psyllium, marshmallow
Digestion	Papaya, peppermint
Digestive Disorders	Safflower, peppermint, ginger, papayaDiuretic Juniper berries, parsley, uva ursi
Dizziness	Yellowdock, dandelion, chaparral
Drug Withdrawal	Dandelion, licorice
Earaches	Lobelia, hops, valerian
Ear Infection	Golden seal; garlic oil (put in ear)
Eczema	Comfrey, burdock, echinacea, chaparral yellowdock
Emphysema	Lobelia, mullein, comfrey (can be taken together); stop smoking

Energy (Lack of)	Ginseng, bee pollen, ginkgo, royal, jelly, gota kola, green additives (barley green, wheat grass, chlorella); clean the colon and the blood; vitamins C and B-complex
Epilepsy	Skullcap, fennel, lobelia
Eye Problems	Bayberry, eyebright
Fasting	Spirulina, licorice; fruit and vegetable juices; food additives (green drinks)
Fever	Peppermint, fresh garlic, rose hips, echinacea
Fibroid Tumors	Red raspberry, don quai; taheebo, chaparral and red clover
Foot Problems	Comfrey foot soak, comfrey and paul d'arco; don't wear tight shoes
Flu	Golden seal, echinacea, peppermint tea and lemon (together)
Fractures	Comfrey, horsetail, slippery elm
Gall Bladder	Golden seal, dandelion, peppermint, buckthorn, comfrey
Gas	Ginger, peppermint, fennel
Glaucoma	Eyebright, alfalfa, fenugreek
Gout	Burdock, safflower
Grey Hair	Horsetail, kelp, oat straw
Gums	Black walnut, comfrey, myrrh
Hair Growths	Horsetail, alfalfa; massage scalp
Hair Health	Alfalfa, sage, Kelp, horsetail
Halitosis (bad breath)	Myrrh, chlorophyll; clean colon
Hangover	Capsicum, wood betony, echinacea, skullcap
Hay fever	Bee pollen, cayenne, alfalfa
Headache	Chamomile, valerian, fenugreek and thyme (together)
Heat (excess body)	Aloe vera, mint herbs (spearmint or peppermint)

Heart	Garlic, cayenne pepper, hawthorn; clean blood, CoQ10
Heartburn	Peppermint, sasparilla, papaya, fennel
Hemorrhage (internal or external)	Cayenne, golden seal
Hemorrhoids	Uva ursi, shepherd's purse
Hepatitis	White oak bark, dandelion, cayenne
Hernia	Red clover, chaparral, clean colon with herbs (aloe vera, senna, etc)
Herpes	Golden seal, black walnut, myrrh
High Blood Pressure	Garlic, cayenne, ginseng, golden seal
Hoarseness	Bayberry, mullein, licorice
Hormone (female)	Dong quai, damiana, blue cohosh, black cohosh
Hormone (male)	Ginseng, saw palmetto
Hyperactivity	Valerian, hops, skullcap; if children are hyperactive stop feeding them sugar
Hypoglycemia	Dandelion, licorice, safflower
Immune System	Golden seal, fresh garlic, echinacea, vitamins A, C, and E (rose hips)
Impotence (erectile dysfunction)	Ginseng, licorice, zinc, arginine, yohimbe, horny goat weed, muira puama
Infection	Echinacea, golden seal
Infertility	Red raspberry, blue cohosh (together)
Inflammation	Echinacea, comfrey, slippery elm
Insect bites	Echinacea, black cohosh
Insomnia	Chamomile, skullcap, catnip, valerian
Insulin	Golden seal (it stimulates the pancreas to produce insulin)
Intestine	Acidophilus
Itching	Yellowdock, plantain, herbal oil

Jaundice	Dandelion, wood betony
Kidneys/Urinary tract	Marshmallow root, juniper berries. Uva ursi: watermelon or cranberry juice
Lactation (decrease)	Parsley, sage
Lactation (increase)	Blessed thistle, marshmallow
Liver	Barberry, Dandelion, Vitamin D
Longevity	Ginseng, ginko, gota kola
Low blood pressure	Cayenne, dandelion, garlic
Lungs	Mullein and Lobelia (together) comfrey, fenugreek; herba santa
Lupus	Dandelion, yellowdock; red clover
Lymphatic system	Echinacea, yellowdock; chaparral and red clover (together); eat less animal product
Memory	Ginkgo, gota kola
Menopause	Dong Quai, black cohosh, false unicorn, blessed thistle
Menstrual Cramps	Red raspberry, chamomile, peppermint
Menstrual Problems	Red raspberry
Mental fatigue	Gingko, ginseng
Migraine Headaches	Chamomile, lobelia
Morning Sickness	Ginger root, peppermint
Motion Sickness	Peppermint, skullcap, catnip, valerian
Mouth Problems	Aloe Vera, golden seal
Mucous	Bayberry, Mullein, golden seal, echinacea; eat less animal products
Muscle cramp	Comfrey, dandelion, alfalfa
Muscle Spasms	Oat straw, lobelia, catnip
Multiple Sclerosis	Lobelia, hops, valerian
Nails	Horsetail
Nausea	Catnip, peppermint

140

Nervous Disorders	Skulcap, catnip, hops, valerian; reduce sugar intake; C and B vitamins
Nightmares	Skullcap, hops
Nose Congestion	Peppermint, spearmint, eucalyptus
Odors (Body)	Chlorophyll
Pain	Chamomile, valerian, wild lettuce; comfrey and mullein (together);
Pancreas	Golden seal, uva ursi
Parasites	Black walnut, herbal pumpkin, fresh garlic, pumpkin seeds
Poison Ivy	Mullein, yellow dock
Perspiration (promote)	Ginger, hyssop, sage
Pregnancy (during)	Red raspberry
Prostrate Problems	Golden seal, pumpkin seeds, ginger; Herbal Pumpkin
Psoriasis	Burdock, chaparral, dandelion Sasparilla; clean colon
Relaxers	Chamomile, hops, valerian, skullcap
Rheumatism	Burdock, alfalfa
Ringworm	Black walnut, golden seal
Sarcoidosis	Mullein and lobelia (together); echinacea and passion flower (together); also clean colon
Senility	Gota kola, ginseng, ginkgo
Senses (enhance)	Ginseng, kelp, any nervine herbs (e.g. hops, skullcap)
Sexual Depressant	Skullcap, hops; keep colon clean; eat lots of green vegetables (mostly raw); eat no animal products
Sexual Stimulant	Ginseng, saw palmetto, damiana (together)
Sexually Transmitted Diseases	Golden seal, echinacea, red clover (all can be taken together)
Shock	Cayenne, lobelia

Sickle Cell Anemia	Dandelion (liver and blood), aloe vera or senna (colon cleanser), and chaparral or echinacea (blood purifier) (together)
Skin (Dry)	Chickweed, dandelion, horsetail. Chamomile, yellowdock, chaparral, red clover, and olive oil can be used externally and internally; also evening primrose oil and wheat germ oil as well as vitamins A and E are good for the skin
Skin (oily)	Horsetail, burdock, aloe vera, dandelion, golden seal, red clover; vitamins A and E are good for the skin
Smoking Habit	Catnip, skullcap, peppermint
Spasms	Catnip, Blue cohosh, lobelia
Spinal Meningitis	Golden seal, lobelia
Spleen	Dandelion, golden seal
Stomach Cramps	Chamomile, peppermint, slippery elm
Stomach Problems	Papaya, peppermint;
Stress	Skullcap, chamomile, hops, valerian; Vitamins C and B-complex
Sugar Habit	Dandelion, licorice
Teeth	Comfrey, black walnut
Throat Soreness or Irritation	Golden seal, cayenne, garlic, licorice extract
Tonsillitis	Echinacea, golden seal
Toothache	Cloves, lobelia, mullein and comfrey (together)
Thyroid	Kelp, irish moss
Ulcers	Cayenne, golden seal, myrrh
Uplift Spirits	Ginseng, blue cohosh; oil of rose, rosemary, or lavender (inhale or apply topically)
Uterus/Ovaries	False unicorn, red raspberry, don quai

Vaginal Douche	Marshmallow, slippery elm, uva ursi
Vaginal Infection	Red raspberry, golden seal
Vaginal Soreness	Aloe vera gel (applied topically)
Wart	Mullein, chaparral
Water Retention	Uva Ursi, cornsilk, parsley
Weight Gain	Chamomile, alfalfa, ginseng, golden seal
Weight Loss	Spirulina, chickweed, and cascara sagrada (together)
Yeast Infection	Acidophilus, black current, eat no animal products.[3]

The third phase of detoxing is with enemas and colonics. Please refer to the chapter on elimination. While fasting, enemas or colonics should be taken daily. Coffee and wheatgrass enemas are great during this cleansing period. The final phase includes saunas, steamrooms, and hot baths with Epsom salt.

Let's conclude this chapter by discussing the little c, cancer, which has so many people afraid. Cancer is a scavenger disease; it lives on waste in the body. If we simply starve the cancer cells they would die. If we had one bowel movement daily we could reduce colon cancer by 33 percent. We could have one bowl movement daily, if we added 13 grams of fiber in our diet.

Exercise reduces breast cancer by almost 20 percent. Unfortunately, cancer is big business in America. The average patient will spend $175,000 on surgery, chemotherapy, radiation, and hospitalization. The medical industry plays with the figures of their success. If diagnosed early radiation and chemotherapy have a success rate of 75 percent, if you only look at three years. If you look at five years or greater the success rate drops to 15 percent. I don't know why they even use surgery, chemotherapy, and radiation when not diagnosed in time. Because my mother was diagnosed in the latter stages, she never should have received surgery, chemotherapy, and radiation. She should have received like all cancer victims the following nutrients to build her immune system.

Apricots

Acidophilus	Flax Seed Oil	Vitamin A	Chlorophyll
Beta carotene	Germanium	Vitamin B complex	Aloe vera
Calcium	Inositol	Vitamin C	Amygdalin/Laetrile
Chromium	Iodine	Vitamin D	Astragalus
Coenzyme Q 10	Manganese	Vitamin E	Cat's Claw
Copper	Potassium	Vitamin K	Echinacea
Fish Oils	Selenium	Zinc	Esiac
Garlic	Gingko Biloba	Ginseng	Green Tea
Iscador		Maitake mushroom	Silymarin
Turmeric	Squalene	Ukraine	Tomatoes
Soy Products	Lycopene	Shark Cartilage	Tribalene

These are just some of the nutrients you need if your immune system can no longer destroy cancer cells. Look at all food and cosmetic products to see if they contain Isopropyl alcohol. This is considered a major contributor to cancer and should be removed from your house. Many Americans who have been blessed with healing want to resume the diet that almost killed them the first time. It reminds me of a back sliding Christian. Many Americans were not aware there are alternatives to doctors, drugs, and surgery. There are also alternatives to hospitals. The insurance industry calls them "alternatives" and will make it difficult for you to use your insurance to pay for them.

In the following chapter, we will provide you with these "alternative" treatment centers, which we feel should be considered first.

HEALING RESOURCE CENTERS

The Bible reminds us in Hosea 4:6, "My people suffer from of a lack of knowledge." Many of us did not know there are other ways to treat illness beside surgery and drugs. Many of us have never visited a naturopath, chiropractor, herbalist, colon therapist, or other natural healers. It is even more difficult for most Americans to identify natural healing centers.

The other major challenge is whether your insurance will pay for these centers. Many of them have been able to position themselves with insurance companies to become acceptable, but in the worst case scenario you have to ask yourself how much are you really worth? Are you willing to use your money to save your life? I would strongly recommend that you become more selective about your insurance or HMO. If your HMO does not allow you to receive service from a holistic healing center you may need change.

These centers offer a number of resources, which include non-toxic medicines, metabolic nutritional programs, tissue cleansing, minerals, vitamins, amino acids, herbs, enzymes, chelation therapy, colon therapy, immunotherapy, acupuncture, massage, saunas, steam rooms, pH balancing, large cell therapy, and detoxification. In addition, most have educational classes so when you leave the center you will be empowered to maintain your new lifestyle.

Listed below are just a few of the hundreds of holistic treatment centers available. I strongly encourage that before you visit another hospital you visit one of these centers.

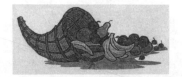
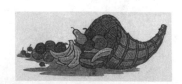

Center for Holistic Life Extension
482 West Ysidro Blvd.
San Ysidro, CA 92713

The Oasis Hospital
4630 Border Village Road
San Ysidro, CA 92173

The main location is Tijuana, Mexico

Holistic Herbal Health Center
RR 1 Wembley
Alberta, Canada TOH350

Uchee Pines Institute
30 Unchee Pines Road
Seale, AL 36875

Better Life Research Center
P.O. Box 238
Canton, CT 06019

Village of Natural Healing
14144 Verona Rd.
Marshall, MI 49068

The Optimum Health Institute
6970 Central
Lemon Grove, CA 91945

The Optimum Health Institute
265 Cedar Lane
Cedar Creek, TX 78612

Creative Health Institute
918 Union City Rd.
Union City, MI 49094

Suluki Wellness and Spa Center
215 Sunset Road
Willingboro, NJ 08046

Center for Alternative Medicine
Harvard Medical School
Beth Israel Hospital
330 Brookline
Boston, MA 02215

Center for Women's Health
Columbia University
630 W. 168th Street
New York, NY 10032

The Center for Alternative Medicine
University of Texas at Houston
7000 Fannin
Houston, TX 77030

National Center for Complimentary
and Alternative Medicine
P.O. Box 8218
Silver Spring, MD 20907

The Christal Center
394 Lake Avenue South
Duluth, MN 55802

Foundation for the Advancement of
Innovative Medicine
485 Kindermack Road
Oradell, NJ 07649

American College for Advancement in Medicine
23121 Verdego Drive, Suite 204
LaGuna Hills, CA 92654

The Atkins Center
152 E 55th Street
New York, NY 10022

The Block Medical Center
1800 Sherman Ave.
Evanston, IL 60201

Health Center Located in Tijuana Mexico
The Triad Medical Center
4600 Kinetz Ke Lane
Reno, NV 89502

HEALING CENTERS

University Health Clinic
5312 Roosevelt Lane
Northeast Seattle, WA 98105

Wellness Center
380 Brinkby Ave.
Reno, NV 89509

A Women's Time
2067 Northwest Love Joy
Portland, OR 97209

Center for Natural Medicine
1330 South East 39th Ave.
Portland, OR 97214

The Revici Life Center
200 W. 57th Street
New York, NY 10019

The Helios Health Center
4150 Darley Ave.
Boulder, CO 80303

The American Metabolic Institute
555 Saturn Blvd.
San Diego, CA 92154
Also a facility in Mexico

The Schachter Center for
Complimentary Medicine
2 Executive Blvd.
Suffern, NY 10901

The Simone Protector Cancer Center
123 Franklin Corner Road
Lawrencedale, NJ 08648

Solstice Chronical Associates
2122 N. Craycroft Road
Tucson, AZ 85712

Wellness Center
3601 Algonquin Road
Rolling Meadows, IL 60008

The Advanced Medicine and Research Center
1000 Cordova Court
Chula Vista, CA 91910
Also have a center in Tijuana Mexico

All Life Sanctuary
P.O. Box 2853
Hot Springs, AR 71914

Christian Brothers
151-47 18th Ave.
Whitestone, NY 11357

Wellspring Center for Natural Healing
2226 Black Rock Turnpike
Fairfield, CT 06432

Wellspring West
1639 Jackson Rd.
Ashland, OR 97520

Hippocrates Health Institute
1443 Palmdale CT.
West Palm Beach, FL 33411

Naples Institute for Optimum
Health and Healing
2329 Ninth St. North
Naples, FL 34103

Ann Wigmore Institute
P.O. Box 429
Rincon, Puerto Rico, 00677
USA 787-868-6307

St. Helena Wellness Center
1000 Trancas
Napa, CA 94558

McDougall Wellness Center
P.O. Box 14039
Santa Rosa, CA 95402

Cancer treatment Centers of America

As you can see several of these sites have their healing centers in Tijuana, Mexico. I strongly recommend Tijuana. They have excellent healing centers. It is also unfortunate that many Americans have to cross the borders to Canada and Mexico because not only is medicine cheaper, but there is an abundance of healing centers, and the availability of herbs and drugs that have not been approved by the FDA, but have shown in numerous studies to have been successful in healing.

The last chapter concerns the group suffering the most in America. The Lord reminds us, "What you do to the least of these, you also do unto me."

THE HEALTH LEGACY OF SLAVERY AND RACISM

I saved this chapter for last because I am very concerned that this population has the worst medical record. There's a popular phrase that when White America catches a cold, Black America suffers pneumonia.

As an advocate of optimal health, I can't help but be concerned about the following statistics and trends. African Americans are 12 percent of the population, but have the highest incidence of prostate cancer in the world. African American males have a 50 percent greater chance than White males to have prostate cancer, and 181 per 100,000 African American males will have prostate cancer. One in three African American males suffer from high blood pressure, versus one in six Whites. African Americans have a 20 times greater chance than Whites of suffering with kidney failure. Twenty-eight percent of all dialysis patients are African Americans. Diabetes is the third leading killer among African Americans, while it is the sixth leading killer among Whites. Ten percent of African Americans have diabetes, but once they become 55 years of age, 25 percent of African Americans will suffer from diabetes.

Thirty percent of all pancreatic cancer patients are African Americans. Forty percent of American women who have fibroids are African Americans. Interestingly, African women have little incidence of fibroids due to a plant based diet. This confirms fibroids are not genetically driven, but result from an animal based processed food diet. Black women have a 400 percent greater chance of suffering from heart disease than White women. AIDS is the number one killer for African American males 25-44, and is the number two killer for African American women.

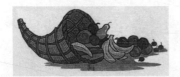 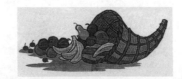

African Americans purchase 38 percent of the cigarettes and 39 percent of the alcohol. There are 288 African American smokers per 100,000, in comparison to 158 Whites per 100,000. The lung cancer death rate for African American males is nearly 54 percent higher than for White males.

Heart disease is the number one killer of African American women, claiming 42 percent of this population. Obesity is a problem for 53 percent of African American women. African American babies are twice as likely as White babies to die before their first birthday: 14.7 deaths per 1,000 live birth vs. 6.1.

African Americans are affected by infertility 1.5 times more often than Whites. High blood pressure is twice as common among African Americans as Whites. One-third of African American have high blood pressure. Some studies estimate at least 75,000 African Americans die annually of manageable diseases.

To me the most dismal statistic, is that African Americans males have a life expectancy of only 66 years, White males and African American females reach 73, and White women live to 79.[1] There are 1.3 million African American women or one in ten who are widows. Fifty-four percent of African American women age 65 and older are widows. African American males are expected to die immediately after receiving their first social security check. They die 13 years before White women. There are 21 underdeveloped countries that have a longer life expectancy than African American males. There is a health crisis in the African American community that must be addressed.

How can a people who developed the laws of medicine with Imhotep thousands of years ago be in such poor condition? How can a people possess the world record in the

100 meters and the marathon, male and female, be in such poor condition? How can a people who were brought to America for slavery because they had great energy, health, and physique be in such terrible condition?

Let's start with the legacy of slavery. The south is considered the "stroke belt." The states include Kentucky, Louisiana, Mississippi, North Carolina, South Carolina, Alabama, Arkansas, Florida, Georgia, Tennessee, and Virginia. They have the greatest incidence of heart disease and stroke in the African American community. During slavery, African Americans were forced to eat the worst food available. Pork was used at every meal, and every part of the pig was used, including the guts, which are called "chitlins." It was during this era that African Americans were forced to be as creative as they could with the worst food provided. While soul food may taste very good it is not good for you. Soul food primarily consists of pork, a lot of fat, fried food, and pounds of sugar.

Oftentimes, you hear the Black community, "I'm going to grease." Unfortunately they mean that literally. The food they are consuming is full of grease. Another phrase you hear is, "Girlfriend can sure burn"; they mean that literally. Black folks like their meat well done. Unfortunately, the longer you cook it the less enzymes are available.

Another phrase you hear is, "She is a healthy sister." A healthy sister is an overweight sister, therefore females that are unhealthy are skinny, and need to visit mama to put some meat on their bones. The average dress size for African American women is a 16. Obesity is five percent greater among African American men and ten percent greater among African American women. The latter group exercises less than the three other groups. Thirty percent of African American women suffer with fibroids. This is three times the rate of white women.[2]

Doctors are quick to recommend surgery and unfortunately many women wait until they're bleeding to make a decision. A better approach would be to eliminate dairy products which have casein (glue) and implement a raw diet, herbs, enemas, colonics, and fasting. The process is longer, requires more effort from the patient, but is cheaper and more beneficial for the body.

As a vegetarian, it has been a major challenge eating in the Black community. I've been to some soul food restaurants where pork was in everything, including the corn. I've seen sweet potatoes where there was more sugar and butter than sweet potatoes. Many times, waiters have told me when I asked was there pork in the beans and greens, they said yes but only for seasoning and you can eat around it. They didn't know that if it is in there for seasoning than it is throughout the entire pot and impossible to eat around.

If you ever visit the African American community on a typical corner will be a storefront church, liquor store, barbecue shop, and a gas station. On some corners they may have two of the above and missing one of those businesses. Liquor stores and barbecue shops dominate the African American community. The body cringes when it has to consume ribs and whisky simultaneously.

I had the privilege of speaking in the Hamptons, a very affluent suburb outside of New York City. It is home to Steven Speilberg and the rich and famous. I thought McDonald's was everywhere. In the Black community fast food chains abound. McDonald's is in Africa, China, Japan, Australia, but not in the Hamptons. This primarily White affluent community does not want their children to consume fast food, which is fried. They want their children to go to delis and consume fresh meats, with fresh produce on wheat bread. Do you know how much effort it takes to have a community void of fast food chains?

I'm also impressed with neighborhoods that have organized to make their communities dry—void of liquor. In the African American community there are few dry neighborhoods. Unfortunately, there have been major efforts by churches but they were fought, not just by the liquor stores primarily owned by foreigners, but fought by the African American residents, who said no one including God can take away their liquor.

Can you imagine an African American community with no liquor stores? Can you imagine an African American community that does not sell pork? Can you imagine an African American community that does not sell fried foods? The Bible reminds us, "Call those things that do not exist as if they were," "Now faith is the substance of things hoped for, the evidence of things unseen." The African American community needs to claim that vision.

Have you ever visited a grocery store in the African American community? It will make you cry. With over 100 different fruits and vegetables that God provides, for some reason in African American stores you see less than ten. I've been to some stores where the only fruit available were bananas, oranges, and apples. The only vegetables were onions and potatoes. What makes it worse, is not only is there less variety, but the quality of the produce is horrendous, and the price is higher than in the White community.

One-third of the African American community live below the poverty line in contrast to 10 percent of the White community. African Americans only earn 61 percent of white income. Twenty-five percent of African Americans lack health insurance.[3] Why should the community that has the greatest number of people living below the poverty line and has a lower income spend more for food and other expenses? God is not pleased with this. Unfortunately, many African Americans who are aware of the disparity drive miles to the suburbs in order to secure red leaf lettuce, broccoli, avocados, mangos, and the other 100 fruits and vegetables other communities take for granted. African Americans must have cars because public transportation will not take them to certain communities.

There have been numerous studies documenting the disproportionate percentage of toxic waste sites near or in the African American community. This is not an accident. The contamination of the soil and the water from these toxic waste sites has been disproportionately borne by the African American community.

As affirmative action continues to be dismantled around the country, there have been a declining percentage of African Americans admitted into medical school, graduating, and returning to the African American community. While the African American population is 12 percent, less than two percent of the doctors are African American and only four percent of the nurses.[4] The problem worsens as HMO's continue to dominate health care in America. Many African Americans doctors are not selected to the HMO pool of doctors.

Many African Americans who, before HMO, had an African American doctor with whom they were pleased no longer have access to them due to racism.

In Cincinnati, African American were 38 percent of the orthopedic surgeons and not one was accepted in any Cincinnati HMO.[5] African Americans are being held hostage by a force outside of itself dictating who will provide health care and making African Americans pay for the service.

Another problem is Black patients often receive less quality medical care. According to Medicare statistics, African Americans are 3.6 times more likely to undergo amputation on lower limbs compared to Whites. Black prostate cancer patients are twice as likely to have their testicles removed than Whites. The most scandalous example of unjust medical treatment for African Americans was published in the New England Journal of Medicine, February 1998. This report shows conclusively that race and sex of a patient independently affect how doctors manage chest pain complaints. In this landmark study by Dr. Kevin Schulman and others, actors of various races and sexes were put on video with identical medical complaints, and were presented to doctors as patients. The result was that the doctors intervened with the gold standard diagnostic tests of cardiac catheterization for White male patients but not for Black male patients.[6]

This is another illustration of the legacy of racism that is affecting the African American community. It has been said that racism contributes to stress. It is a major culprit and is a driving force for strokes, high blood pressure, and heart disease. The two major causes for stress in the African American community are discrimination and poverty. Numerous studies have pointed out that the last thing that a

White person would want to have happen to them is to be
Black living in America. Diane Elliot and other researchers
on race relations have illustrated to the White community
with a blue-eye green-eye study as one example. Blue-eyed
students were discriminated against and even though they
knew it was a simple exercise that would end in less than an
hour, the amount of stress that it placed on them was cata-
strophic. If you multiply that by a lifetime you begin to get
some idea of what it is like for an African American who
makes the same amount of income as a White American and
is denied an apartment, mortgage, employment, car note,
business loan, etc.

The other driving force is poverty. It is very difficult
living in a capitalistic materialistic society and watching tele-
vision and observing people living in mansions while you
are living in squalor. Some of the living conditions of African Americans, whether it's in housing developments in the
north or chanteys in the south, are not fit for humans. Many
African Americans have lack of access to health care and
only visit an emergency room when there is a crisis. Many
African Americans do not visit a doctor until the pain has
become so severe there was no other choice. Unfortunately,
the options are greatly reduced. An ounce of prevention is
still the best cure.

From a genetic perspective, 70 percent of African
Americans cannot properly digest cow's milk. Most African
Americans don't have the enzyme lactase to digest it properly. We mentioned earlier the negative consequences of
consuming cow's milk, this is further exacerbated in the African American community.[7]

Because of the larger amount of melanin that African
Americans possess, they become more addicted to nicotine,

caffeine, and cocaine.[8] These three drugs have become severe in the African American community. Sixty percent of all inmates are there due to drug related crimes.

One of the concerns that I have in the church community, is when the pastor or ministerial staff reads the names of the sick and shut in list. Immediately after the announcement, they mention the church is serving ham and eggs after the first service and "chitlins" after the second service. I have two concerns. The first is obvious that the pastor or minister have not made the connection between diet and health care. The church is contributing to the sick and shut in list with this terrible diet.

Just as you can look at many doctors and not see a healthy, vibrant, energetic doctor, the same applies to many pastors. There's a joke in the Black Christian community that you can tell when a person is saved if they are overweight. They have given up on the flesh and are developing their spirit. That is not biblical—your body is the temple of God.

The second concern I have is when the sick and shut in list is read what are we going to do about it? Are we going to lay hands on these people? Are we going to have intercessory prayer? Is there any power in the congregation to address the sickness taking place in the church? You listen to some reports and it seems hopeless. I see a lot of powerless churches that do not believe in healing scriptures.

The African American community has 85,000 churches; unfortunately many of them are entertainment and containment churches. They sing, dance, and shout but are powerless. The Black community needs more liberation churches.

These churches stand on the Bible and believe that God is a healer.   Liberation churches have pastors who teach their congregation to stand on God's word, in spite of the doctor's prognosis. Liberation churches do not allow liquor stores and barbecue shops to be their neighbors. They develop healing centers for their communities.

EPILOGUE

Satan I'm taking back my health. I know you come to steal, to kill, and to destroy, but my Savior came to give me life and to give me life more abundantly. He wants me to prosper in all things, including my health as my soul prospers. I will drink more water. I will eat fruit and salad daily. I will take vitamins and herbs. If I don't eliminate daily I will take an enema or colonic. I will exercise at least three times a week. My health no longer belongs to the doctor, it belongs to me. My body houses the Holy Spirit. I am fearfully and wonderfully made. To God be the glory in Jesus' name, Amen.

*P.S. Please give a book to someone who needs healing. To my mother I regret that you left too soon. I miss you dearly, but I know **where** you are, I know **who** you are with, and I will see you again!*

FAITH & HEALING SCRIPTURES

These Scriptures are to be meditated not just read. Upon meditating, create a confession and read daily.

Faith Scriptures

Joshua 1:8 * Mark 11:23-24 * Matthew 9:27-29
Mark 9:23 * 2nd Corinthians 5:7 * Romans 4:17
Romans 10:17 * Hebrews 11:1

Healing Scriptures

2nd Kings 20:5 * Psalms 30:2 * Psalms 103:3 * Psalms 107:2
Isaiah 53:5 * Jeremiah 8:22 * Jeremiah 30:17 * Jeremiah 33:6
Mark 5:21-43 * Mark 6:13 * Mark 16:18 * Luke 17:11-14
Hebrews 13:8 * James 5:13-15 * 1st Peter 2:24

References

Chapter Three

1) Centers for Disease Control. 1999 Annual Report. Dr. Atkins' Health Revelations 1999 Editions. Roizen, Michael. *Real Age*. New York: Harper Collins, 1999.
2) Steward, H. Leighton. *Sugar Busters*. New York: Ballantine Books, 1999, p. 19.
3) Robbins, John. *Diet For a New America*. Tiburon California: H.J. Kramer, 1987, pp 356–358.
4) Centers for Disease Control.
5) Malkmus, George. *Why Christians Get Sick*. Shippensburgh: Destiny Image, 1995, p.7.

Chapter Four

1) Pescatore, Fred. *Feed Your Kids Well*. New York: John Wiley 1999, p.17.
2) Malkmus, George. *God's Way to Ultimate Health*. Shelby, North Carolina: Hallelujah Acres, 1995, pp. 85-86.
3) Diamond, Harvey and Marilyn. *Fit For Life*. New York: Warner Books, 1985, pp. 43, 95. Robbins, p. 155.
4) Gaynor, Mitchell. *Dr. Gaynor's Cancer Prevention Program*. New York: Kensington, 1999, pp. 7–8, 91, 97.
5) Pescatore, pp. 18–40.
6) Roizen, p. 212.
7) Diamond, W. John. *Definitive Guide to Cancer*. California: Future Medicine, 1997, p.107.

Chapter Five

1) Jantz, Gregory. *21 Days to Eating Better*. Grand Rapids: Zondervan, 1998, p. 85.

2)   Kunjufu, Jawanza. *Developing Positive Self-Images and Discipline in Black Children.* Chicago: African American Images, 1984, pp.73–74.
3)   Bell, G. Textbook of Physiology and Biochemistry. New York: Ballentine, 1954, pp. 167–170.

Chapter Six

1)   Wright, Keith. *A Healthy Foods and Spiritual Nutrition Handbook.* Philadelphia: Health Masters, 1990, p. 27.
2)   Dorian, Terry. *Health Begins in Him.* Lafayette: Hantington House, 1995, p.143.
3)   Wright. p. 28.
4)   Ibid. p. 21.
5)   Kirshman, John. *Nutritional Almanac.* New York: McGraw Hill, 1979.

Chapter Seven

1)   Eades, Micheal and Mary. *Protein Power.* New York: Bantam 1998, p.5.
2)   USDA Agriculture Handbook no. 456. McDougall, John. The McDougall Plan. Clinton: New Win, 1983, p. 99.
3)   Robbins. pp. 367, 372.
4)   Ibid, p. 315.
5)   Eades, p. 39.
6)   Ibid, p. 310.
7)   Atkins, Robert. Dr. Atkins' New Diet Revolution. New York: Avon, 1992, p. 46.
8)   Eades, pp. 9,46–48.
9)   Atkins, p. 196.
10)   Journal of the National Cancer Institute Vol. 51 no. 6.
11)   Robbins, p. 265.
12)   Cancer Research 35:3374, 1975.

13)   Ibid.
14)   Advances in Cancer Research 32:237, 1980.
15)   Robbins, p. 195.
16)   Ibid. p. 192.
17)   Ibid. pp. 193–194.
18)   Wright, pp. 84–85.

Chapter Eight

1)   Know – About Publications. Harrisburg, PA. 1975.
2)   The Story of Beef. The American Meat Institute. Chicago.
3)   Robbins, pp. 63–71.
4)   Ibid. p. 380.
5)   Pesticides Monitoring Journal 2:140–152, 1969.
6)   Dorian, pp. 91–92.
7)   Robbins, p. 247.
8)   Roizen, p. 185.
9)   Robbins, pp. 156–157.
10)   Ibid. p. 157.
11)   Ibid. p. 157.
12)   Dorian, p. 105.

Chapter Nine

1)   Asante, Molefi. *Ancient Egyptian Philosophers*. Chicago: African American Images, 2000, pp. 41-54.
2)   Journal of Longevity. Vol. 5, No. 3, 1999, p. 21.
3)   Robbins, p. 150.
4)   Money Magazine, October 1999, p. 48.
5)   New England Journal of Medicine, January, 1999.
6)   USA Today. " Divvying Up Healthcare", December 1, 1999, p. 29A.
7)   Mindell, Earl. *Prescription Alternative*. Los Angeles: Keats, 1999, p. 3.
8)   Ibid. p. 328.
9)   Ibid. pp. 285–288.

10)   Ibid. pp. 289–290.
11)   Ibid. p. 277.
12)   Ibid. p. 277.
13)   Dr. Robert Atkins' Health Revelations. Volume VI, November 9, September, 1998, p. 5.
14)   Journal of Longevity, Vol. 5, No. 3, 1999, p. 32.
15)   Health Alert, November 1999, p. 16.
16)   Mindell, p. 54.
17)   Journal of Longevity, p. 33.
18)   Journal of Family Practice, June, 1999.
19)   Smythe, Benjamin. Killing Cancer: The Jason Winters Story. Las Vegas: Vinton Publishing, 1980, p. 47.

Chapter Ten

1)   Archives of Internal Medicine, October 25, 1999, 159:2273.
2)   Anton, Rein. "Reversing Heart Disease." Brecher, Harold. *Consumers Guide to Chelation Therapy.* Herndon: Healthsavers Press, 1993.
3)   Wright, pp 59–67.

Chapter Eleven

1)   Walker, Marcellus. *Natural Health for African Americans.* New York: Warner Books, 1999, pp. 4–5. Ebony Magazine. May 1999 pp 159- 163. Citizen Newspaper. June 17, 1999, p. 13. Centers for Disease Control.
2)   NDIGO, "Heart Disease Now No. I Killer of Black Women," February 10, 1999, p. 5.
3)   U.S. Statistical Abstract, 1999.
4)   Emerge Magazine, September 1999, p. 36.
5)   Ibid. p. 38.
6)   Emerge Magazine, October 1999, p. 32.
7)   Afrika, Llaila. *African Holistic Health.* Silver Spring: Sea Island Information Group, 1989, p. 3.

Dr. Jawanza Kunjufu is available for
sermons
retreats
seminars
conferences
Bible study

Please contact 773-445-0322 (Telephone)
or
773-445-9844 (Fax)
or
ritask@africanamericanimages.com (E-mail)
or
African American Images
1909 W. 95th Street
Chicago, IL 60643

NOTES

NOTES

NOTES

NOTES

NOTES

NOTES

NOTES

NOTES

NOTES

NOTES

NOTES

NOTES

NOTES

NOTES

NOTES